SJ
ALLE ZEIT WACH
1842

W. Eicher (Editor)

F. Kubli †, V. Herms (Coeds.)

Plastic Surgery in the Sexually Handicapped

With 125 Figures and 22 Tables

Springer-Verlag Berlin Heidelberg New York
London Paris Tokyo

Professor Dr. med. Wolf Eicher (Ed.)

Frauenklinik
Diakonissenkrankenhaus Mannheim
Akademisches Lehrkrankenhaus der Universität Heidelberg
Speyerer Straße 91–93
D-6800 Mannheim 1

Professor Dr. med. Fred Kubli † (Coed.)

Klinikum der Universität Heidelberg
Frauenklinik
Voßstraße 9
D-6900 Heidelberg 1

PD Dr. med. Volker Herms (Coed.)

Abteilung Gynäkologie und Geburtshilfe
Kreiskrankenhaus
Krankenhausstraße 46
D-8765 Erlenbach/Main

ISBN-13: 978-3-642-73567-7 e-ISBN-13: 978-3-642-73565-3

DOI: 10.1007/978-3-642-73565-3

Library of Congress Cataloging in Publication Data.
Plastic surgery in the sexually handicapped / W. Eicher (eds); F. Kubli, V. Herms (coeds.).
Papers presented at a satellite symposium of the 8th World Congress for Sexology, June, 1987, Heidelberg, Germany. Includes index.
ISBN-13: 978-3-642-73567-7
1. Generative organs–Surgery–Congresses. 2. Breast–Surgery–Congresses. 3. Sexual differentiation disorders–Surgery–Congresses. I. Eicher, Wolf. II. Kubli, F. (Fred). III. Herms, V. (Volker). IV. World Congress of Sexology (8th: 1987: Heidelberg, Germany)
[DNLM: 1. Breast–surgery–congresses. 2. Genitalia–surgery–congresses. 3. Sex Differentiation Disorders–surgery–congresses. 4. Surgery, Plastic–congresses. WJ 700 P715 1987]
RD584.P52 1988 617'.463–dc19 DNLM/DLC 88-24974

Softcover reprint of the hardcover 1st edition 1989

Typesetting: Brühlsche Universitätsdruckerei, Giessen
Offsetprinting: Saladruck, Berlin. Bookbinding: Lüderitz & Bauer, Berlin
2121/3020-543210 – Printed on acid-free paper

Preface

Sexual medicine is an interdisciplinary subject. Special knowledge of normal and disturbed sexuality is expected of general practitioners, gynecologists, dermatologists, urologists, specialists in internal medicine, neurologists, psychiatrists, and psychotherapists. Sexual dysfunctions may occur in connection with organic lesions or as psychosomatic phenomena. They are brought to the practicing physician's attention by the patient either directly or in the form of factitious symptoms. The disturbed sexual function generally causes suffering and so motivates the patient to consult a physician. Psychosomatic aspects are thus very much to the fore.

In a significant number of cases, however the disturbances stem from a physical-functional handicap which not only affects the patient's general personality but also has a direct adverse effect on sexual function. The physical defect leads to disturbances of the body-image, and so can cause impairments in the sexual sphere both directly and indirectly.

The diseases which result in sexual handicap and which can be treated by reconstructive surgery were examined and discussed at an international satellite symposium of experts on the occasion of the 8 th World Congress for Sexology in June 1987. The papers presented at this symposium have been collected and edited in this volume.

Breast surgery, including congenital anomalies and reconstruction after amputation, genital malformations, from congenital anomalies in the vaginal area and of the penis through to the deformities of intersexuality and aplasia of the vagina, changes due to genital prolapse in women, the lost penis syndrome and impotence with vasosurgical and prosthetic remedies, and genital transformation in the case of transsexualism (both male-to-female and vice versa) are the main topics of interest to plastic, pediatric, and vascular surgeons as well as to urologists and gynecologists with regard to surgical technique. They are, however, of equal importance to all other physicians who are involved in sexual medicine.These include general practitioners, specialists in internal medicine, andrologists, gynecologists, urologists, pediatricians, and – not least – psychiatrists and psychotherapists.

Our special thanks are due to Springer-Verlag, publishers of international repute who enjoy a high standing in the field of medicine. Their support, particularly with regard to the many illustrations, has been extremely generous and their editorial staff have given us valuable assistance.

Mannheim, August 1988 Prof. Dr. Wolf Eicher

In memoriam Prof. Dr. Fred Kubli †

Introduction to The International Satellite Symposium of the 8th World Congress for Sexology on Reconstructive Surgery in the Sexually Handicapped
By Fred Kubli †

Ladies and Gentlemen,

It is a great pleasure for me to welcome you to this symposium on reconstructive surgery in the sexually handicapped. I must say it is a special honor for me to co-chair this meeting with Prof. Eicher, who is one of the two presidents of the World Congress of Sexology and has done an enormous amount of work to promote sexual medicine at the regional, national, and international level.

Sexual handicap is an extremely wide field, one, I think, that has no limits. We are all probably in agreement that the basic problem is a psychological one. However, the subject of our meeting today is not this essential problem – we are going to deal with technical questions. If you want to have good results in psychological terms, you also need good techniques and good technical skills. There is no good medicine without good techniques.

To which groups is this subject of interest? The field is so wide, and so technically diverse that all kinds of disciplines are involved. It involves gynecological and neurological surgery, pediatric surgery, vascular surgery, and of course, above all, plastic surgery. It also involves urology and diagnostic radiology. These are the disciplines which are actively involved in the treatment of sexual handicap.

However, there is another, maybe larger, audience which needs to know what can be done: this comprises general practitioners, general gynecologists and urologists, general pediatricians and neurologists, psychiatrists and psychotherapists, and of course all sexologists – in other words, all those who are confronted in their consulting rooms with sexual problems. This meeting is mainly directed towards this audience to demonstrate what can be done today in terms of relief and reduction of sexual handicaps.

† This introduction was given by Prof. Dr. Kubli who, sadly, died before production of this book was complete.

We are extremely pleased and honored to have such outstanding experts from all over the world as guest speakers, and we are very thankful and very much obliged to them for their participation.

Heidelberg, 15 June 1987

Contributors

Altwein, J. E.
Bartsch, G.
Borruto, F.
Bouman, F. G.
Davydov, S. N.
Debrovner, C.
Denil, J.
Eberle, J.
Eicher, W.
Hentz, V. R.
Herms, V.
Homoki, J.
Klika, T.
Kubli, F.
Laub, D. R.
Laub, D. R. II
Michal, V.
Müller, A.
Payan, F.
Rochet, Y.
Schreiter, F.
Strömbeck, J. O.
Wagenknecht, L. V.
Woodhouse, C. R. J.
Yachia, D.

Contents

Part 5: Genital Transformation

Part 6: Penis Prosthesis in Impotence

Part 7: Vascular Impotence

Part 1: Breast Surgery

Surgical Correction of Breast Deformities

J. O. Strömbeck

Plastikkir. Kliniken Sabbatsbergs Sjukhus, Box 6401, 11382 Stockholm, Sweden

A deviation in the size or configuration of the breasts from what is regarded as normal for the ethnic group to which a woman belongs may give rise to considerable psychological problems, with effects on self-esteem and a feeling of deficient womanhood. Besides psychological problems, pronounced hypertrophy will give rise to somatic symptoms caused by the weight as such. Surgical correction of such deformities is a very rewarding task.

Reduction Mammaplasty

Many techniques for the reduction of oversized breasts have been developed since the 1920s. The ideal procedure should give a breast of adequate size and natural shape, and it should preserve sensitivity and function (Fig. 1). My personal preference in surgical technique is illustrated in Fig. 2, which shows a preoperative planning of nipple transposition and skin flaps, and a resection from the areas superior, lateral, and inferior to the areola-carrying medially based pedicle, which is connected to the major part of the remaining gland.

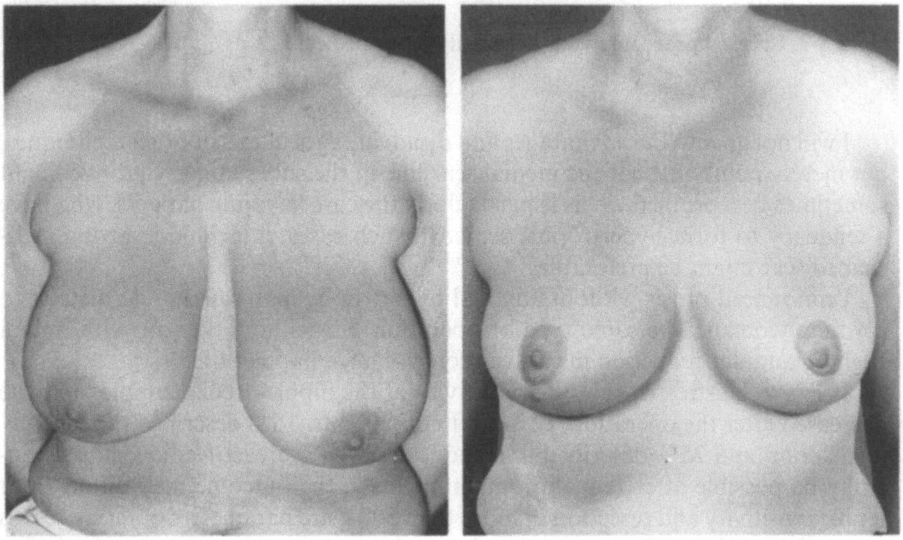

a b

Fig. 1 a and b. Macromastia **a** before and **b** after surgery

Plastic Surgery in the Sexually Handicapped
Eds.: W. Eicher/Kubli/Herms

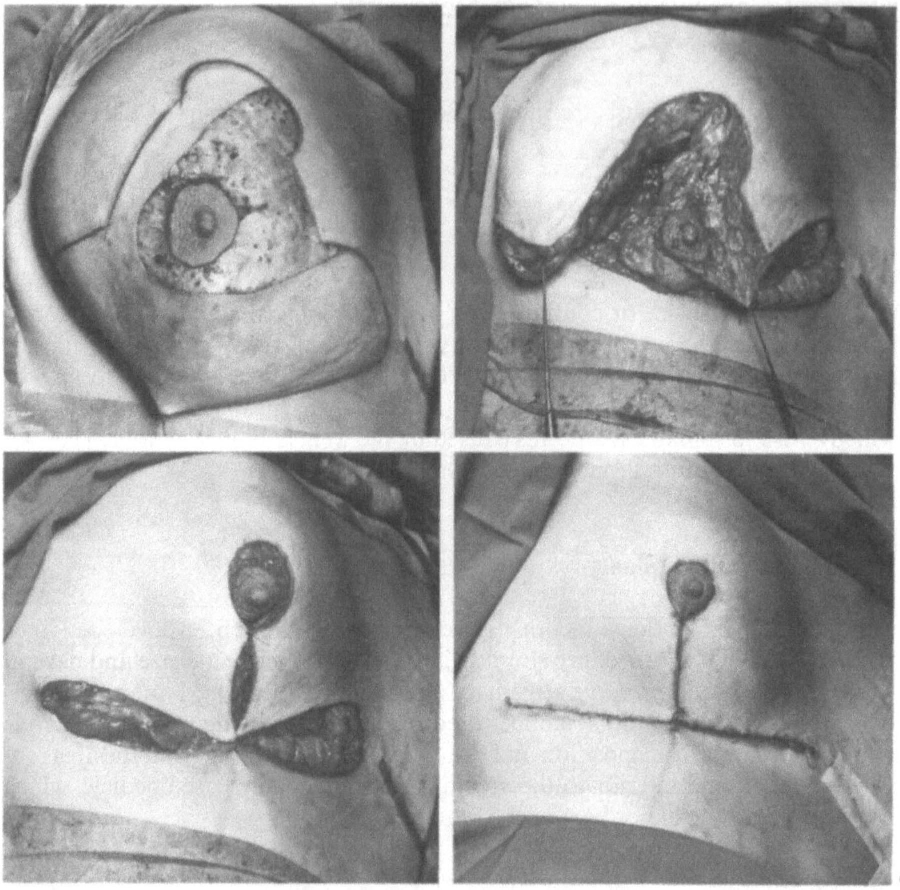

a b c d

Fig. 2 a–d. Surgical procedure with a medially based pedicle

I will not go into the advantages and disadvantages of this or other techniques, but merely point out that the medial scar line in the submammary groove might sometimes be a problem. This is particularly the case in young patients, who have a tendency to form hypertrophic scars. In such cases, a technique giving in L-shaped scar might be preferable.

Pronounced ptosis without any real hypertrophy may cause great distress to a young woman. The same type of operation but without any, or with only a slight, glandular reduction may give such women a happier life.

It has to be stressed that the sensitivity of the nipple-areola complex may be decreased after the operation. In a group of patients, 15% described the sensitivity as poor, and 25% described it as reduced. Even if breast-feeding should generally be possible after reduction mammaplasty, the outcome may differ. Poor nipple sensitivity and resection of more than 500 g are parameters pointing to less successful nursing. Of a group of patients who had nursed both before and after the operation, half reported equally good breast-feeding before and after, a quarter reported worse, and a quarter better nursing capacity after the operation. As preoperative information, I tell the patient that she has a 50% chance of good breast-feeding, which is probably to underestimate the probability.

Augmentation Mammaplasty

The possibilities for augmenting a small breast have increased tremendously during the past 30 years through the development of increasingly inert prosthetic materials. Implanting a submammary prosthesis is a simple way of building up a suitable breast volume (Fig. 3).

The still unsolved problem is how to avoid a capsular contracture, which gives rise to an unnatural hardness of the breast. Many possible reasons for this contracture have been discussed, such as hematoma, foreign body reaction, and subclinical infection. What we know is that inflatable prostheses and submuscular implantation cause less contracture than gel prostheses and subglandular implantation. A consistently soft and natural breast may be expected in 30%–80% of all patients, depending on the technique used. The incision can be axillary, periareolar, or in the submammary fold. The pocket for the prosthesis is made subglandularly or submuscularly. The prosthesis can be of silicon gel, inflatable, or a combination of both.

My personal preference is to make a submuscular pocket from an incision in the submammary groove. Today, I mostly use a double-lumen prosthesis with a core of silicon gel and an outer lumen filled with saline. It has to be stressed that the pocket should be made large enough, and that the caudal circumference of the muscular pocket should be left open.

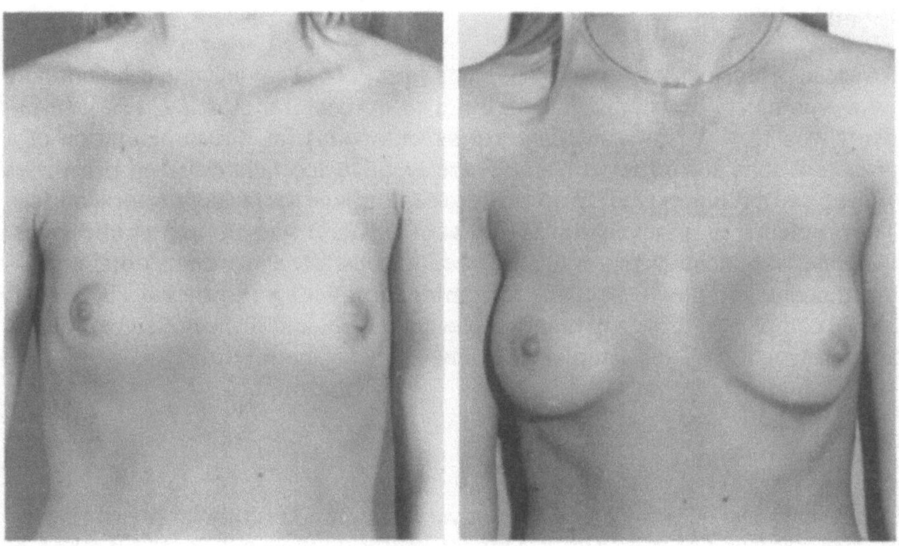

a b

Fig. 3 a and b. Micromastia **a** before and **b** after surgery

Breast Asymmetries

Breast asymmetries are common (Fig. 4). Depending on the situation, a reduction of the enlarged side or an augmentation of the small side may be made, or an augmentation on one side and a reduction on the other. Of course, there are cases where a reduction has to be made on both sides.

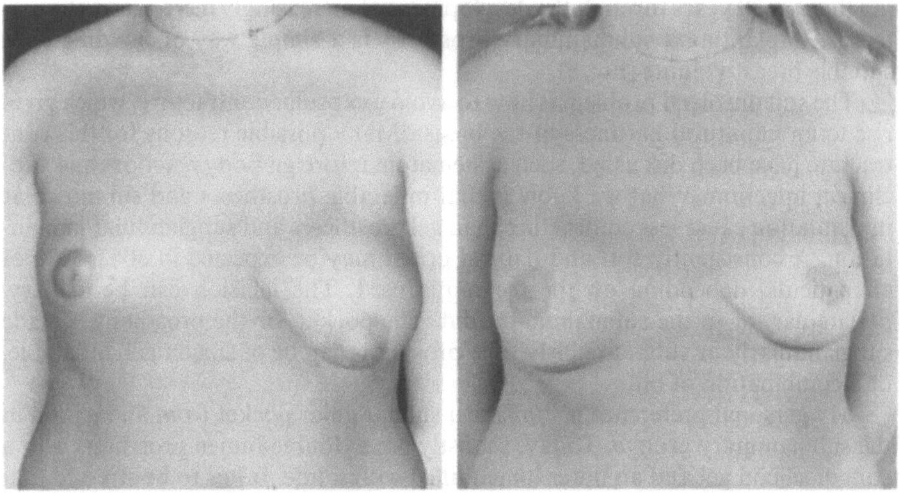

a b

Fig. 4 a and b. Breast asymmetry **a** before and **b** after surgery

Poland's Syndrome

A special problem is presented by patients with Poland's syndrome, who not only have a complete unilateral amastia but also no pectoral muscle (Fig. 5). In patients who have a reasonable layer of subcutaneous fat, the implantation of a prosthesis may solve the problem. There are also specially designed prostheses with an extra filling extending upwards to camouflage the lack of pectoral muscle. The problem is in principle similar to that of a patient who has had a radical mastectomy. In patients with very little subcutaneous fat, a latissimus dorsi musculocutaneous flap has to be made in combination with a prosthesis. The areola-nipple complex in these patients is of the male type, and if the patient so wishes, a reconstruction of this complex may add to the cosmetic effect.

Tubular Breast

A further breast deformity which is not very uncommon is tubular breast (Fig. 6). If such breasts are oversized, a conventional reduction will be the method of choice. In smaller tubular breasts, the shape will be remarkably improved by re-

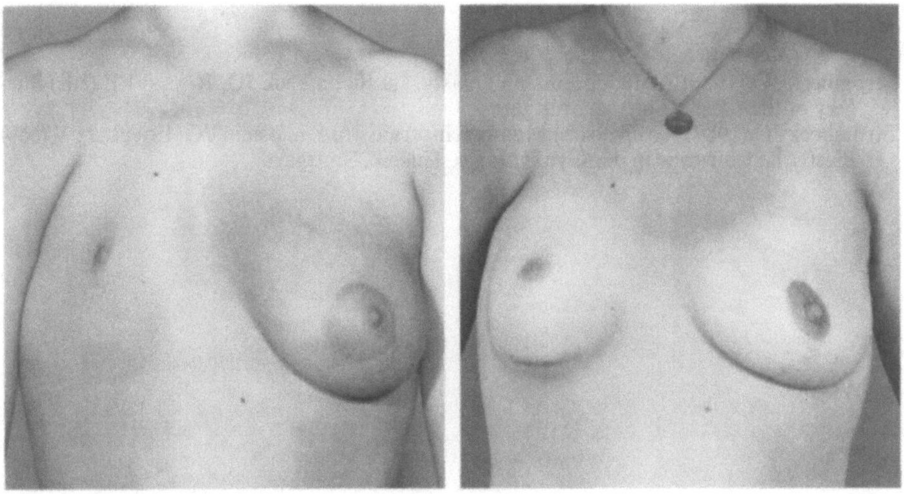

a b

Fig. 5 a and b. Poland's syndrome **a** before and **b** after surgery

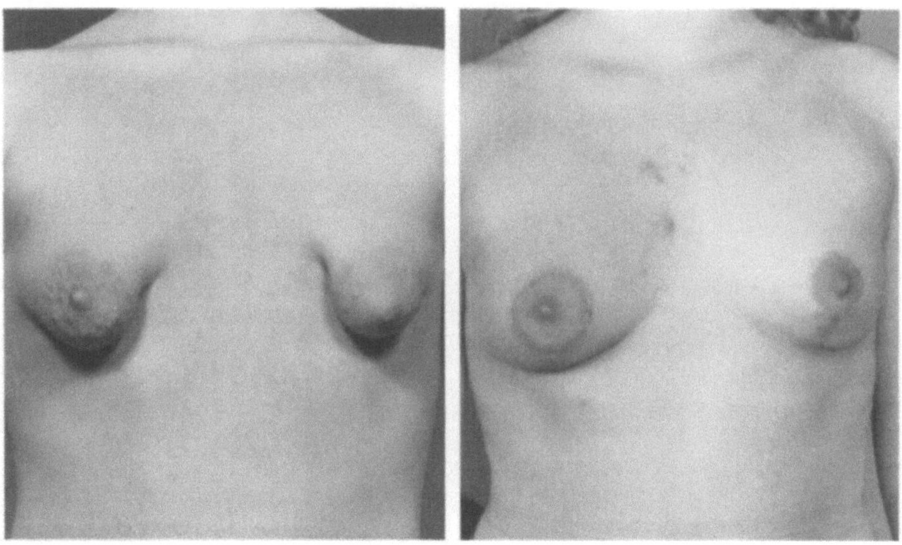

a b

Fig. 6 a and b. Tubular breast **a** before and **b** after surgery

duction of the often very extended areola in combination with a wide undermining of the skin in all directions, extending to the base of the breast and well below the submammary fold.

In summary, it could be said that plastic surgery offers techniques to deal with different types of breast deformities, and that this type of operation is a most satisfying field in plastic surgery.

References

Strömbeck JO (1986) Reduction mammaplasty. In: Strömbeck JO, Rosato FE (eds) Surgery of the breast. Thieme, Stuttgart

Strömbeck JO (1987) Kosmetische Mammachirurgie. In: Knapstein PG, Friedberg V (eds) Plastische Chirurgie in der Gynäkologie. Thieme, Stuttgart

Breast Reconstruction After Mastectomy

F. Kubli [1], V. Herms [2], and A. Müller [1]

[1] Universitäts-Frauenklinik, Voßstraße 9, D-6900 Heidelberg, FRG
[2] Gynäkolog. u. geburtshilfliche Abteilung, Kreiskrankenhaus, 8765 Erlenbach, FRG

I would like to consider some of our experiences with skin expanders in breast reconstruction. The Department of Obstetrics and Gynecology in Heidelberg is a center of primary treatment of breast cancer, with almost 400 cases of primary therapy every year. About 30–35% of these are breast-conserving operations, and the rest are of necessity conventional; in these latter cases, we offer reconstruction. This has been our procedure for more than 10 years, and now, on the basis of a 160-month follow-up of patients with reconstructed breasts and matched controls, we can clearly demonstrate that there is no difference in outcome; i.e., reconstruction certainly does not adversely affect the prognosis of breast cancer patients as far as the survival rate is concerned.

For the last 10 years, our technique has consisted in overexpansion: we introduced an inflatable prosthesis not only under the skin but below the pectoral muscle at primary or secondary treatment, and this overinflation was a one-stage procedure. The results were – at least in part – very good during this 10-year period.

But to return to the skin expander: between August 1983 and April 1987, we used the skin expander in 145 cases, and the whole procedure has already been completed in 122 cases. The expander consists of an inflatable reservoir, into

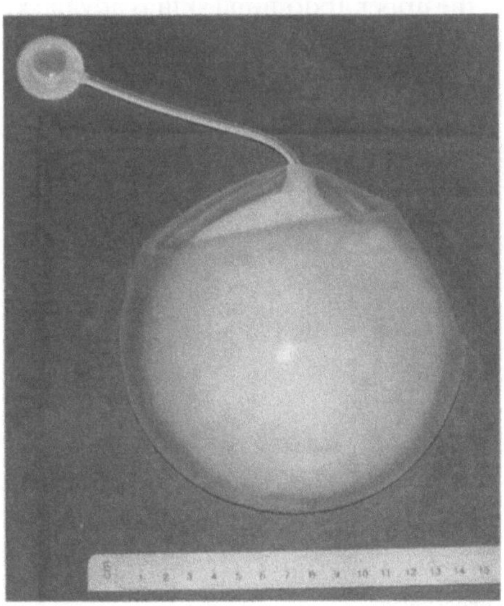

Fig. 1. Skin expander

Plastic Surgery in the Sexually Handicapped
Eds.: W. Eicher/Kubli/Herms

which small portions of the normal saline are filled regularly, week by week, through an axillary valve by transdermal injection (Fig. 1).

The following remarks concern the basic technique. We performed primary reconstruction at the time of breast amputation in 72% of our patients, and for the rest – patients who had been operated on elsewhere or had made the decision later – we did it as a second step. In contrast to Olivari's, our procedure is always a two- to three-stage operation. The first step is the implantation of the expander below the pectoral muscle; additionally of course, the serratus muscle and the external oblique abdominal muscle are used. This submuscular expansion will in general take 2–3 months after implantation, with an average of 2.5 months and a range of 1–4 months. About 3–6 months after the primary implantation, there are three possibilities for the second stage of our procedure. First, the expander can simply be replaced by the final, gel-filled prosthesis. The second possibility, which I will examine in more detail, is to shape a new, reconstructed breast. Finally, in some cases, the previously untouched contralateral breast needs to be adapted for the sake of symmetry; this was done in 61% of our patients. The third stage consists of reconstruction of the nipple and areola. Not all of our patients are keen to undergo this stage, perhaps because so many operations are necessary. We have only done this step in one-fifth of the patients, but we are not being overzealous. It is often reported that the surgeons are more insistent than the patients, most of whom are already glad to have a new breast.

Through overexpansion, the volume is increased so that it is clearly higher than that finally intended, which greatly facilitates further planning. A line is drawn from the projected new areola to the submammary fold, and if there is an overhang of skin, this will be disepithelized and inverted. From this site, one makes the incision to open the submuscular space, where the expander is located. All that remains after discarding the expander is a musculocutaneous sliding flap, with which it is very easy to form a new breast. After insertion of the gel prosthesis, it is very simple to make the new inframammary fold symmetrical to the contralateral one (Figs. 2, 3). In the final stage, the upper abdominal skin is advanced vertically and fixed at the new site, which again is very easy. Some relatively good

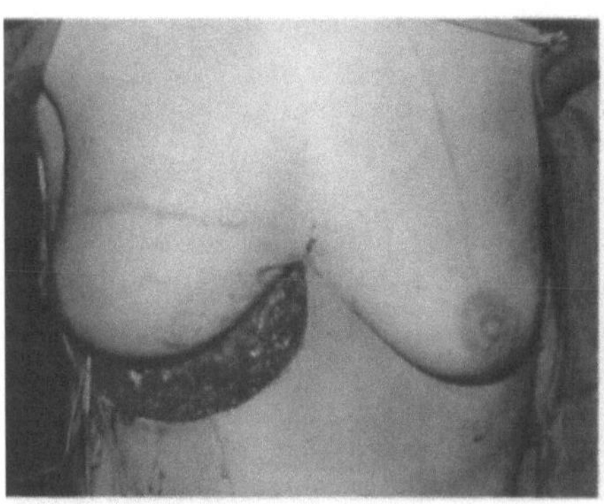

Fig. 2 a and b. Inframammary fold

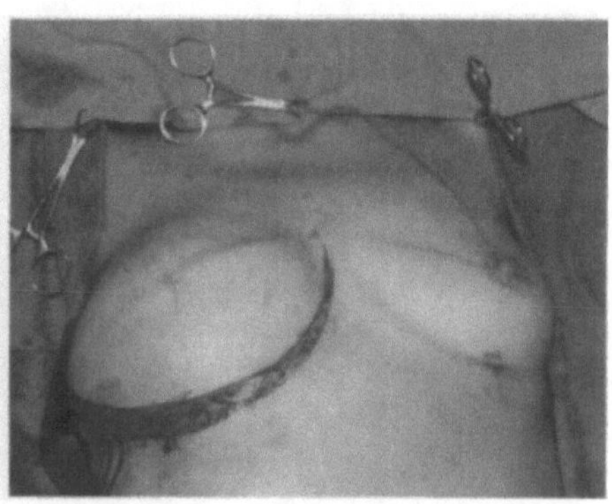

Fig. 3. Inframammary insertion of gel prosthesis

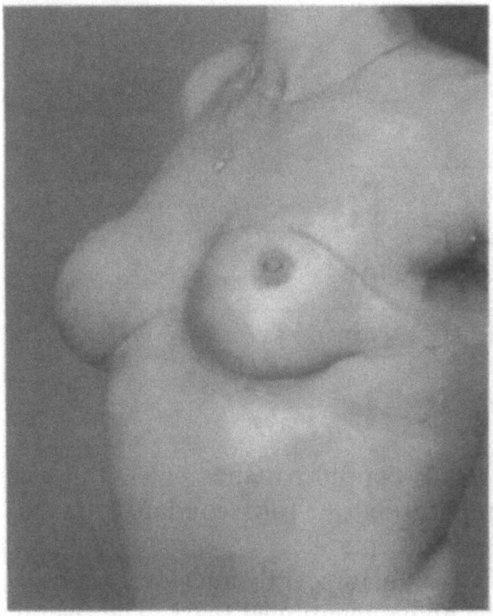

Fig. 4. Postoperative result

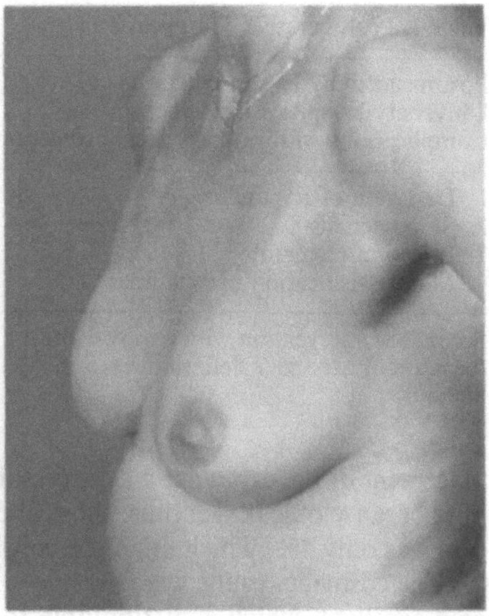

Fig. 5. Postoperative result

early results are shown in Figs. 4, 5. When we begin an expansion, it is not necessarily our intention to alter the contralateral breast; often, this proves to be unnecessary, and we even achieve symmetry without adaptation.

About a year ago, this technique was criticized by Olivari because it involves making a new submammary fold, and I now concede that this criticism was fair: there really are problems with the new inframammary fold. Due to capsular contraction and dislocation of the prosthesis, the scar can be some distance from the true inframammary fold; thus the whole scar is exposed, and the final result is most unsightly. I think it would be wrong to expect all reconstruction to be beautiful.

The overexpanded reconstructed breasts had an average volume of 500 ml, with a range of 200–800 ml. In a relatively small number of cases, we simply replaced the larger expander prosthesis with a smaller gel-filled prosthesis, which also produces symmetrical ptosis, but not the true inframammary fold. Active shaping as outlined above was done in the majority (80%) of our cases.

In mentioning the main complication, I would like to stress that it must be considered scandalous that the companies concerned do not seem capable of constructing inflatable prostheses which last and do not have leaks. The major complication – occurring in 20% of our patients – during the phase of expansion was deflation, leaks of the expanders, which seems to me absolutely disgraceful, bearing in mind the price of the devices.

The rest of the complications would appear to be within the normal range (Table 1). There was skin necrosis in 3% of our patients, infections and hematoma in up to 8%, and major dislocation of the expander in 4%. It is important to underline the fact that although secondary intervention with removal or re-

Table 1. Postoperative complications

Postmastectomy Reconstruction University Hospitals Heidelberg Complications with primary Reconstructions	
1. Deflation of Expander	18/88 = 20,5%
2. Skin necrosis	3/88 = 3,4%
3. Infection/Hematoma	7/88 = 8,0%
4. Major Dislocation of expander	4/88 = 4,6%

Secondary intervention with removal and/or exchange of expander necessary: 9/88 = 10,2% (because of expander deflation $n=5$ (6%).

placement of the expander was necessary in 10% of our patients, in 6% this was only because of leakage; thus, the real complication rate for secondary intervention was only 4%, which might be considered acceptable.

The cosmetic results were evaluated by two doctors. Only a few were considered excellent, which is attributable to the above-mentioned scars. The overall good-or-excellent rate of 60%, however, is acceptable, and I think it is relatively realistic. We had bad results in 10% of our patients, and I think a lower percentage is difficult to obtain.

To summarize the advantages of the expander technique at the present time from our point of view: the first and major advantage is that the implant may be inserted at primary treatment, independent of how radical this treatment is. As an oncologist, one can shape the primary operation according to the stage of the tumor. It is not difficult to insert the expander because the volume is increased later step by step. One cannot expect too much with regard to the final cosmetic result in particular, due to the scar problem. In our opinion, reduction and lifting of the contralateral breast is necessary less often than with conventional techniques. In our experience, capsular contraction is observed with a frequency roughly similar to that seen in other procedures of plastic surgery. However, there is a second problem: the action of the innervated muscular cover often prevents a longer-lasting ptosis. Furthermore, the muscle will retract very slowly even without capsular contraction. But with lack of ptosis – as mentioned above – the problem of visibility of scars arises.

Our present procedure can be summarized as follows. We still do primary or secondary submuscular implantation of the expander, placing it about 1–2 cm below the planned new inframammary fold. We perform an overextension to a volume about one-third greater than that of the contralateral breast. In the second stage, we mainly replace the expander with the final gel prosthesis, trying to avoid creating new scars. If we form a new inframammary fold, we try to do so from an internal approach, which is slightly more difficult for us but is, of course, possible. In most cases, an adaptation of the contralateral breast is in fact still necessary because of the problems outlined above.

Part 2: Genital Malformations

Feminization of Children with Adrenogenital Syndrome Using the Nerve-Sparing Technique: Experience with 25 Girls

J. E. Altwein [1] and J. Homoki [2]

[1] Department of Urology, Krankenhaus der Barmherzigen Brüder, Munich, FRG
[2] Department of Pediatrics, University of Ulm, Ulm, FRG

A number of surgical procedures have been developed for the correction of various degrees of genital masculinization in adrenogenital syndrome (AGS) and related disorders of sexual differentiation. Although sometimes defended with fervor, these procedures are not always applicable in all patients with equally good results (Flach 1977; Fonkalsrud et al. 1977; Glassberg and Laungani 1981; Ringert and Walz 1985; Starinka et al. 1968; Stefan 1966). The goals of these measures are (a) to achieve the closest possible resemblance to the female genitalia, (b) to retain orgasm ability, (c) to make sexual intercourse possible, and (d) to take into consideration the emotional situation of the child and her parents.

The most frequent cause of ambiguous genitalia in the newborn is AGS, with a frequency of 1 in 5000–15000 births. This is followed by the various forms of gonadal dysgenesis, with a rate of 1 in 25000 (Griffin and Wilson 1986).

The surgical repair should preferably be done in one session, and it includes (a) clitoroplasty, (b) labioplasty, (c) monsplasty, and (d) vaginoplasty. Although vaginoplasty performed early in childhood often requires revision after puberty (Bolkenius and Daum 1977; Rajfer et al. 1982; Ringert and Walz 1985; Spence and Allen 1973), it usually facilitates the clitoroplasty. In order to achieve a correction which will be effective for the entire duration of childhood, it is desirable that vaginoplasty be performed by the age of 2 years. The intention is for the child to be able to recognize that she is a girl by the time she develops the faculty of recollection and by the onset of gender identification (about 2.5 years of age; Lewis and Money 1977; Money and Hampson 1955). At this time, the genitalia are clearly visible and of such proportions as to make good and lasting cosmetic results possible. In the event that the family is psychologically unstable and the mother in particular has difficulties accepting her child as a girl, the feminization procedure should be done earlier (Lewis et al. 1970).

Since von Neugebauer performed a cut-back vaginoplasty and clitoral amputation in 1908, a variety of clitoroplasties have been introduced, i.e., clitoral recession, corporal plication, clitoral relocation, and clitoral reduction (Allen 1985, Perlmutter 1986). The last of these is performed as a nerve-sparing procedure and is combined with reconstruction of the mons and introitus (Praetorius 1981). Our experience in operating on 25 girls with AGS using this approach is reported below.

Plastic Surgery in the Sexually Handicapped
Eds.: W. Eicher/Kubli/Herms

Patients and Method

Between 1980 and 1986, 26 girls were subjected to nerve-sparing feminization genitoplasty as described by Praetorius (1981). A technique of remarkable similarity was recommended by Snyder et al. (1983). Of the patients treated, 25 had virilized external genitalia due to conadrenal hyperplasia; of these, 23 had a 21-hydroxylase deficiency, 1 had an 11-β-hydroxylase deficiency, and 1 had maternal virilization. One individual with mixed gonadal dysgenesis is not included in this report. The degree of virilization was classified according to Prader (1954) (2); 64% had a Prader 4-type virilization. Of the 25 girls, 17 (68%) were below 3 years of age, i.e., before gender identification, and 4 had previously had a clitoral recession, their ages at the time of definitive correction being 4, 6, 12, and 16 years, respectively. It is of note that one girl aged 3.5 years with a Prader 5 AGS initially had a wrong, male karyotype, requiring gender reassignment.

Operative Technique

Nerve-sparing feminizing genitoplasty as described by Praetorius (1981) has been reported in detail previously (Altwein and Walz 1983) and the surgical principles have been reiterated by Snyder et al. (1983); therefore, a few surgical details will suffice (Figs. 1–4). The clitoris is approached dorsally, the skin being divided almost at the ventral commissure of the labia majora. In dissecting the cheeks of the glans, its size is reduced. The cheeks are left attached to the triangular foreskin to form the lining of the vaginal introitus (Fig. 4). After exposing the clitoral nerve, the crura are severed. The glans remains with a dorsal pedicle (the neurovascular bundle) and a ventral pedicle (the urethral plate; Merberger (1967). The suspensory ligament of the clitoris, with its superficial and deep dorsal veins, is maintained. The principle of Fortunoff et al. (1964) is used in the vaginoplasty, and that of Perlmutter (1986) in the monsplasty.

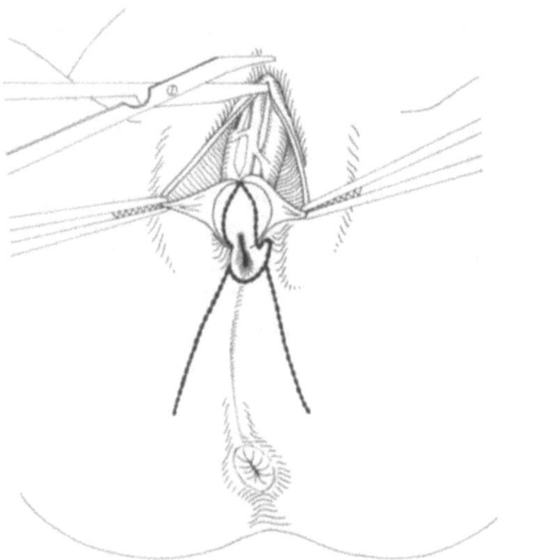

Fig. 1. The skin of the clitoral phallus is divided dorsally. Vessels and nerves lying above and below Buck's fascia are indicated. *Dotted lines* illustrate the direction of the further incisions

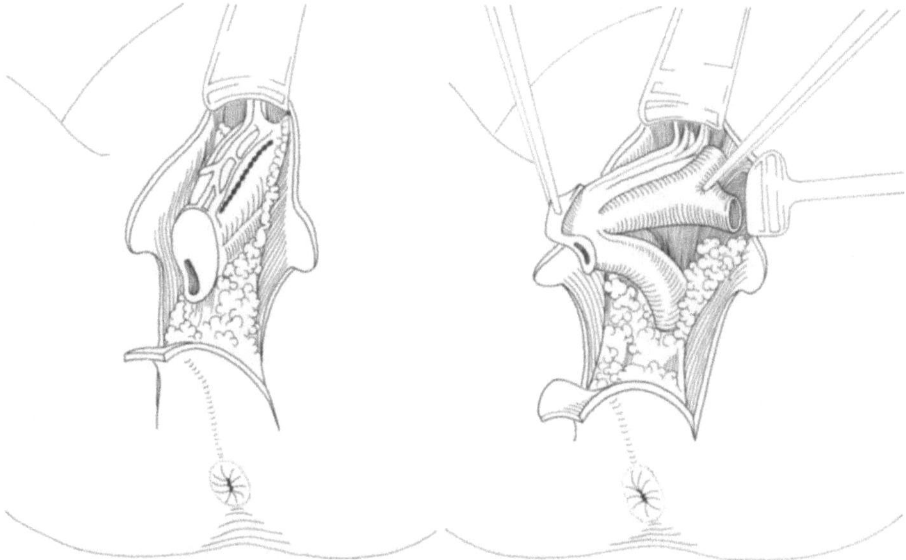

Fig. 2a, b. The crura of the corpora are severed just below the pubis, after identification of the pudendal nerve. The distal portions of the corpora are not entirely freed from the glans in order to provide a higher degree of stability. The nerve and blood supply of the glans remains intact within the dorsal bridge of tissue and the urogenital canal

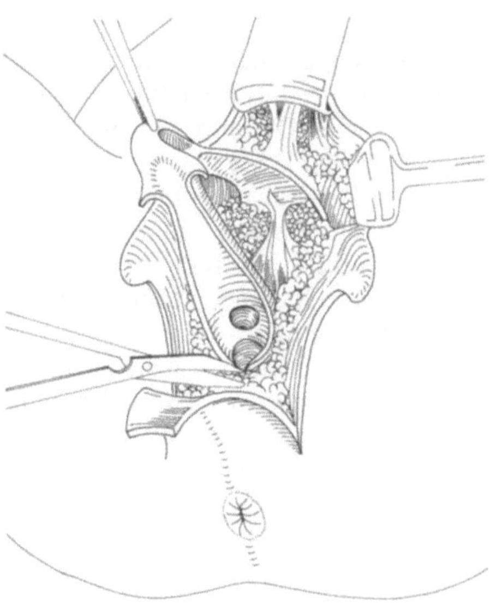

Fig. 3. The urogenital canal is divided until the vaginal orifice appears

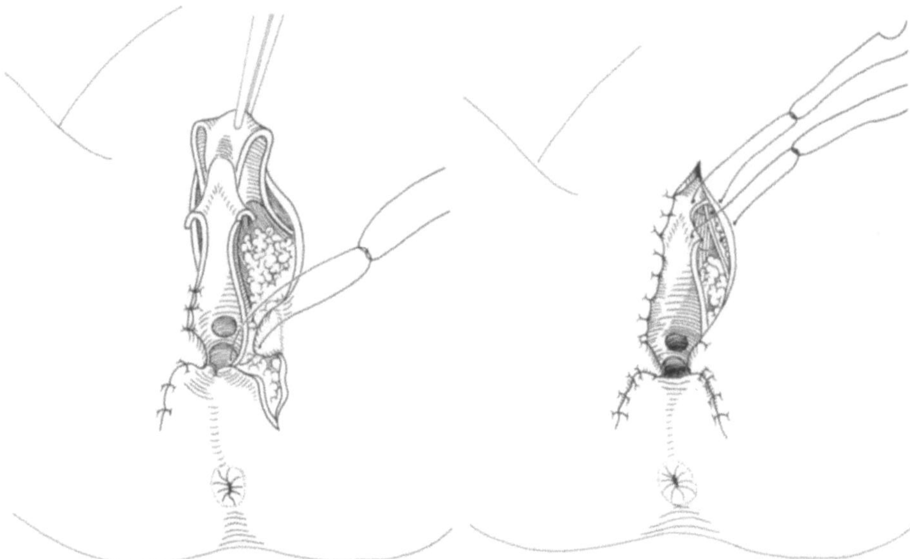

Fig. 4. a The freed sides of the glans and foreskin are folded inward and sutured to the vaginal introitus. The perineal flap is fixed to the vagina. The dorsal bridge of tissue containing nerves and vessels is placed under the anterior commissure of the labia majora. **b** If the vaginal introitus does not lie too proximal and the perineum is not too high (Prader 2 and 3), the cheeks of the glans can be sutured into the angle at the base of the perineal flap, as not all the material is required

For the Prader 5 AGS, the same method was used; the major portion of the skin forming the pseudoscrotum was discarded. The urethra is spatulated from the sulcus coronarius proximally to the perineal muscles. Definitive vaginoplasty in the Prader 5 condition is deferred until puberty (Allen 1985).

With the exception of the first six patients, 6-O PDS (Polydioxamone Sulfate; Ethicon, Hamburg, FRG) served as suture material. Usually, an 8-F silicon catheter was left indwelling until the compression dressing was removed. A well-fitting vaginal tampon was also inserted. After photodocumentation, the girls were discharged between the 8th and 10th postoperative day.

Follow-up control was possible in all 25 patients, with an average of 40 months. At the last examination, the cosmetic appearance was assessed by the authors and the parents. Tactile glandular sensation was evaluated by testing the girls' perception of a pinprick (Barrett and Gonzales 1980). The somatosensory evoked potentials were measured in one girl by Scherb (1987).

Results

One-step feminizing genitoplasty was accomplished in 25 patients with AGS. In two Prader 5 patients, the highly placed vaginal entry prevented exteriorization of the vagina since this maneuver would open the proximal urethra and carries the risk of stress incontinence.

Cosmetic Appearance

In 24 of 25 patients, the female appearance was judged by the parents and the authors to be highly satisfactory. In one of the girls with Prader 5 AGS, the appearance was found unsatisfactory due to the scrotiform vulva; however, the superfluous skin was saved in part for vaginal exteriorization after puberty.

Functional Outcome

With one possible exception, the glans clitoridis had a well-preserved blood supply, which would not be maintained with the ventral pedicle alone (Young 1937). In one 4-year-old girl, the parents consented to a study of the somatosensory evoked potentials via the pudendal nerve as compared with the tibial nerve, which indicated the presence of sensitivity in the former (Scherb, personal communication 1987). When last seen, the introitus measured 14–16 F in the girls 1–6 years of age, 30 F in the 12-year-old, and 36 F in the 16-year-old patient.

Complications

Of the 25 patients, 4 had early complications. A hemorrhage from the corpus cavernosum excision occured in one of the girls with a Prader 5 AGS due to a postoperative rise in blood pressure. The 16-year-old patient had an intraoperative laceration of the rectum due to a narrow, scarred introitus; healing was, however, uneventful. Late complications were observed in 8% of the patients.

Discussion

Various problems have been associated with previously described clitoroplasty techniques. Clitorectomy was widely applied since it is technically easy and produces an acceptable cosmetic appearance; however, because of questions raised about altered erotic responsiveness after amputation, this option is now generally contraindicated (Perlmutter 1986).

The apparent size of the shaft can be reduced by clitoral recession (Schmid 1961) preserving clitoral sensation by relocating the glans. This procedure and the corporal plication technique (Glassberg and Laungani 1981; Stefan 1986) conceal the glans as a result of its size being disproportionate to the surrounding genitalia, and they result in bulging of the shaft during erection.

Procedures involving shaft resection without preservation of the dorsal neurovascular bundle (Dapunt and Marberger 1970; Spence and Allen 1973) will not be likely to achieve a functional status any different to that of the "cosmetic clitoris" described by Jones and Jones (1954) or that achieved by clitorectomy operations.

All forms of virilization are characterized by an enlarged glans, which usually remains concealed under a foreskin synechia during the early years of life. All operations which retain the glans have been reduction techniques, such as dorsal excision or circular ablation of the corona glandis (Huffstadt 1967; Stefan 1966). Other conservative procedures preserving the glans in toto are only done if it does not exceed a particular size, which, however, is never precisely defined; otherwise, the glans is amputated.

Schmidt (1961), Starinka et al. (1968), and Kumar et al . (1974) first gave thought to the innervation of the glans and its dissection. They were instrumental in developing an optimal compromise between function and cosmetic appearance, after the group around Money had demonstrated the importance of performing phenotype correction early in childhood (Lewis et al. 1970; Lewis and Money 1977; Money and Hampson 1955; Perlmutter 1986). Nerve-sparing reduction clitoroplasty in which part or all of the shaft is excised with glans preservation is the most accepted and widely used technique today (Allen 1985; Altwein and Walz 1983; Bartsch et al. 1987; Kogan et al. 1983; Mollard et al. 1981; Praetorius 1981; Rajfer et al. 1982; Snyder et al. 1983).

Since the external alterations are mainly brought about by the hypertrophied clitoris – and since its further growth cannot be predicted with certainty, even with good hormonal regulation – it should be corrected in such a way as to guarantee a normal female appearance, at least up to the time of pubic hair development. Shaft-preserving procedures can only achieve this effect if the enlargement is minimal (Perlmutter 1986; Ringert and Walz 1985).

The usually longitudinally oval glans clitoridis assumes a spherical shape under the influence of androgen. By retaining the dorsal and ventral nerve and blood supply, it is possible to reduce the lateral portions of the glans (Praetorius 1981). This simulates the natural situation better than circular ablation. If the glans is no longer fixed to the corporal stump under the symphysis arch, but is rather developed ventrally, brought in front of the symphysis body, and fixed there in the subcutaneous tissue, the ventral bridge of tissue stretches, and the dorsal bridge can easily be placed under the anterior commissure.

The basic principles of Snyder's (1966) labioplasty have merely been subjected to variation in all the subsequent methods (Bolkenius and Daum 1977; Dapunt and Marberger 1970; Flach 1977). Only Perlmutter (1986) pulled the foreskin folds over the stump of the resected clitoris in a different manner. The foreskin has also been resected. Formation of labia minora is most successful when the clitoris is large and the introitus only minimally altered. In Prader 4 and 5 conditions, the phallic skin is only barely sufficient to completely cover the vaginal introitus newly formed by flap vaginoplasty. The pull-through vaginoplasty of Hendren and Crawford (1969) should be able to solve the labia question alone and optimally. This form of very early vaginal creation has, however, been severely criticized by gynecologists (Dewhurst 1982; Richter 1982); moreover, the cosmetic results achieved are only mediocre. Any vaginoplasty that requires dilatation up to the age of puberty in order to achieve lasting success will adversely affect the psychological development of the child (Bolkenius and Daum 1977).

The immediate and long-term results of the Praetorius technique have been found to be highly satisfactory in 25 children operated on in this way. The cosmetic appearance of the vulva and the preservation of glandular function – as shown by measuring the somatosensory evoked potentials – meet the essential goals of feminizing surgery.

References

Allen TD (1985) Disorders of sexual differentiation. In: Kelalis PP, King LR, Bleman AB (eds) Clinical pediatric urology, vol 2, 2nd ed. Saunders, Philadelphia, p 904

Altwein JE, Walz PH (1983) Urologische Behandlung der Intersexualität. In: Hohenfellner R, Zingg EJ (eds) Urologie in Klinik und Praxis, vol 2. Thieme, Stuttgart, p 1114

Barrett TM, Gonzales ET Jr (1980) Reconstruction of the female external genitalia. Urol Clin North Am 7:455

Bartsch G, Schachtner W, Marberger H (1987) Erhaltung des Gefäßnervenbündels bei der Klitorisreduktionsplastik. Akt Urol 18:96

Bolkenius M, Daum R (1977) Verbesserte Methode zur operativ-plastischen Korrektur der Klitoris bei Pseudohermaphroditismus femininus. Z Kinderchir 20:71

Dapunt O, Marberger H (1970) Die operative Reduktion der vergrößerten Klitoris. Geburtsh Frauenheilk 30:433

Dewhurst J (1982) Surgical treatment of genital tract malformations. In: Richter K (ed) 1. Europäisches Symposium für Kinder- und Jugendgynäkologie 1981. Wissenschaftliche Information Milupa, Friedrichsdorf, FRG, vol 1, pp 237 and 278

Flach A (1977) Die plastische Korrektur des äußeren weiblichen Genitales im Kindesalter. Z Kinderchir 21:168

Fonkalsrud EW, Kaplan S, Lippe B (1977) Experience with reduction clitoroplasty for clitoral hypertrophy. Ann Surg 186:221

Fortunoff S, Lattimer JK, Edson M (1964) Vaginoplasty technique for female pseudohermaphrodites. Surg Gynecol Obstet 118:545

Glassberg KI, Laungani G (1981) Reduction clitoroplasty. Urology 17:604

Griffin JE, Wilson JD (1986) Disorders of sexual differentiation. In: Walsh PC, Gittes RF, Perlmutter AD, Stamey TA (eds) Campbell's urology, vol 2, 5th edn. Saunders, Philadelphia, p 1819

Hendren WH, Crawford JD (1969) Adrenogenital syndrome: the anatomy of the anomaly and its repair. Some new concepts. J Pediatr Surg 4:49

Huffstadt AJC (1967) Surgical correction of female pseudohermaphroditism due to adrenal hyperplasia. Br J Plast Surg 20:359

Jones HW, Jones GES (1954) The gynecological aspects of adrenal hyperplasia and allied disorders. Am J Obstet Gynecol 68:1330

Kogan SJ, Smey P, Levitt SB (1983) Subtunical total reduction clitoroplasty: a safe modification of existing techniques. J Urol 130:746

Kumar H, Kiefer JH, Rosenthal IE, Clark SS (1974) Clitoroplasty: experience during a 19-year period. J Urol 111:81

Lewis VG, Ehrhardt AE, Money J (1970) Genital operations in girls with the adrenogenital syndrome. Obstet Gynecol 36:11

Lewis VG, Money J (1977) The need of early surgical feminization in girls. In: Lee PA, Plotnick LP, Kowarski AV, Migeon CJ (eds) Congenital adrenal hyperplasia. University Park Press, Baltimore, p 463

Marberger H (1967) Zur chirurgischen Behandlung nebennierenbedingter Scheinzwitter. Der Urologe 6:153

Mollard P, Juskiewenski S, Sarkissian J (1981) Clitoroplasty in intersex: a new technique. Br J Urol 53:371

Money J, Hampson JC (1955) Hermaphroditism assignment of sex, change of sex and psychologic management. Bull Johns Hopkins Hosp 97:284

Perlmutter AD (1986) Management of intersexuality. In: Campbell's urology, vol 2, 5th edn. Saunders, Philadelphia, p 1934

Prader A (1954) Der Genitalbefund beim Pseudohermaphroditismus femininus des Kongenitalen Syndroms. Helv Paediat Acta 9:231

Praetorius M (1981) Zur Korrektur des AGS-Genitales bei stärkeren Virilisierungsformen (Prader III–V). Z Kinderchir 33:343

Rajfer J, Ehrlich RM, Goodwin WE (1982) Reduction clitoroplasty via ventral approach. J Urol 12:341

Richter K (1982) Probleme bei der Behandlung der Aplasia vaginae. Round table epilogue. In: Richter K (eds) 1. Europäisches Symposium für Kinder- und Jugendgynäkologie. Wissenschaftliche Information Milupa, Friedrichsdorf, FRG 8:295

Ringert RH, Walz KA (1985) Ergebnisse operativer Therapie der virilisierten Vulva. Akt Urol 16:229

Scherb W (1987) personal communication

Schmidt MA (1961) Plastische Korrektur des äußeren Genitales bei einem männlichen Scheinzwitter. Arch Klin Chir 29:977

Snyder CC (1966) Sex syndromes. Mod Trends Plast Surg 2:285

Snyder HM, Retik AB, Bauer SB, Colodny AH (1983) Feminizing genitoplasty: a synthesis. J Urol 129:1024

Spence HM, Allen TD (1973) Genital reconstruction in the female with the adrenogenital syndrome. Br J Urol 45:126

Starinka L, Stavratjev M, Toman M (1968) Plastic adjustment of female genitals in adrenogenital syndrome. Acta Chir Plast 10:99

Stefan H (1966) Chirurgische Behandlung des äußeren weiblichen Genitales bei weiblichen Pseudohermaphroditen. Z Kinderchir 3:249

von Neugebauer FL (1908) Hermaphroditismus beim Menschen. Klinkhardt, Leipzig, p 431

Young HH (1937) Genital abnormalities, hermaphroditism and related adrenal diseases. Williams and Wilkins, Baltimore

Posterior Hypospadias

J. Eberle and G. Bartsch

Department of Urology, University of Innsbruck, Amichstraße 35,
6020 Innsbruck, Austria

Embryology

Normal male sexual development (Bergoda et al 1962; Jost 1953, 1972) comprises three sequential steps. Starting at the moment of fertilization, genetic sex is established as a result of interactions between genetic material on the autosomes and genetic determinants on the X and Y chromosomes. In the second step, genetic sex is translated into gonadal sex. According to several working models (as e.g. described by Walsh et al. 1974), a male-specific cell surface histocompatibility antigen is responsible for differentiation into an ovary or testis. Germ cells in the male develop in the entoderm of the yolk sack during the 3rd week of fetal life. After migration, they reach their specific location in the primitive gonads. In approximately the 6th week of gestation, the human testis develops rapidly, starting with differentiation of the tubuli seminiferi. In the 9th week, Leydig cells appear, initiating endocrine functioning.

After the establishment of chromosomal sex and the development of gonadal sex, the third step is the transformation of gonadal into somatic sex – the male and female phenotypes. No sex-specific differences are found in the development of the human reproductive tract out of two complete sets of ducts prior to the 7th week of gestation.

Masculine differentiation of the indifferent urogenital tract and external genitalia depends on the secretion and action of three fetal testicular hormones: testosterone, 5α-dihydrotestosterone, and müllerian inhibiting substance (Bartsch et al. 1986; Forest 1975; Frederick and Wilson 1986; Siiteri and Wilson 1974). The last of these suppresses the müllerian ducts and leads to almost complete regression, except for a small cranial portion, the appendix testis, and the lower end, which remains as the prostatic utricle. Testosterone stimulates virilization of the wolffian ducts and induces the development of the epididymis, vasa deferentia, and seminal vesicles. Finally, 5α-dihydrotestosterone induces transformation of the derivatives of the urogenital sinus (Fig. 1).

During the 4th week of gestation, the urorectal septum divides the cloaca, forming an anterior sinus urogenitalis and posterior rectum. Because of the vast developmental potential of the surrounding mesoderm, paired swellings appear on both sides of the cloacal membrane. The two anterolateral swellings fuse, creating the genital tubercle – the primordium of the glans penis in the male and of the glans clitoridis in the female. On the caudal aspect, the urethral and genital folds are formed, separated by the urethral groove (Fig. 2).

Plastic Surgery in the Sexually Handicapped
Eds.: W. Eicher/Kubli/Herms

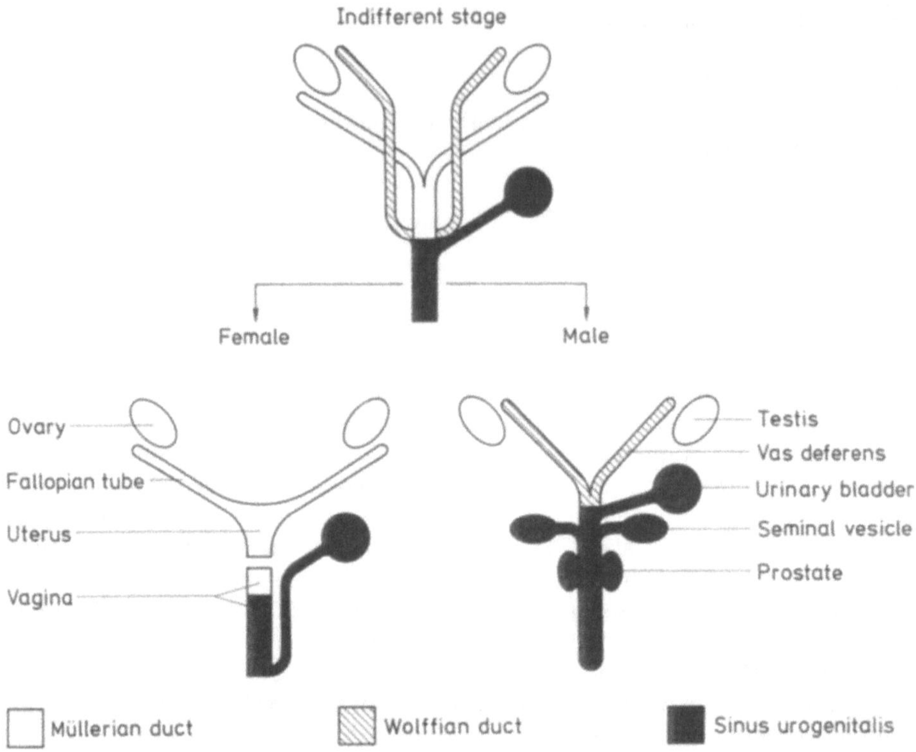

Fig. 1. Sexual differentiation of internal genitalia. (From Tunn et al. 1981)

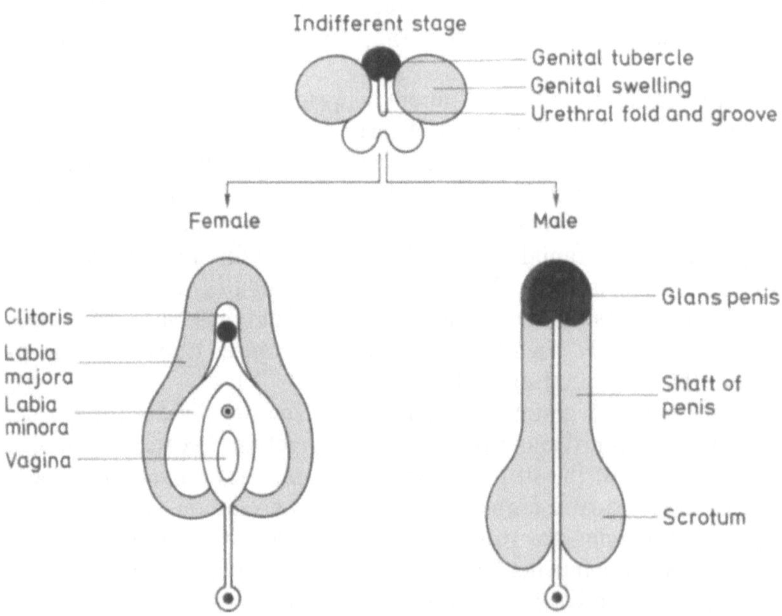

Fig. 2. Sexual differentiation of external genitalia. (From Tunn et al. 1981)

In all of these mesodermal derivatives, 5α-reductase – the enzyme responsible for irreversible conversion of testosterone to dihydrotestosterone – is present, and high endogenic levels of 5α-dihydrotestosterone, necessary for normal differentiation of the external genitalia, are obtained. It may be that less androgen is required for the development of the internal genitalia; this would explain why normal and early sexual differentiation of the internal genitalia can be associated with abnormalities of the external genitalia, as in hypospadias, involving the shaft of the penis and the urethra.

In association with the formation of the phallus, the urethral groove extends to the level of the corona, and the urethral folds close and become progressively fused from the basal to the distal aspect, forming the urethra and the median raphe of the scrotum and penis. The genital swellings merge and migrate caudally, enlarging to form the scrotum at the base of the penis. The glandular urethra is a compound of proliferating ectoderm, which burrows into the glans to meet the penile urethra. Intimately related to the fusion of the urethral folds, the prepuce is formed over the glans penis with a ridge of skin, enclosing the glans circumferentially.

Incomplete coalescence results in various degrees of hypospadias, with the urethral meatus placed ventral and proximal to the normal location on the tip of the glans. A dorsal preputial hood is found around the glans in varying configurations. The undeveloped urethra distal to the displaced meatus consists of fibrous elements, believed to be remnants of urethral mucosa and arrested corpus spongiosum. This persisting mesenchyme (chorda) causes the characteristic downward curvature of the penis. Hypospadias is a common and complex deformity; the posterior type, with the meatus situated perineoscrotally, is found in about 20% of cases. Our interest centers on these disorders of the male phenotypic development.

Diagnostic Procedures

The decision about sex assignment should be made immediately after birth to assure normal psychosexual orientation of the child. Before selecting an appropriate therapeutic modality, it is necessary to make a correct and early diagnosis of the ambiguous genitalia and associated abnormalities, which are difficult to detect.

The first step in the evaluation requires an exact family history, including pedigree analysis (Nowakowski and Lenz 1961; Simpson et al. 1971). There follows a critical physical examination, in particular of the size and shape of the phallus and scrotum, and of the location of the urethral orifice and the presence of a chorda. Chromosomal sex is determined by counting the Barr bodies, karyotyping, or using fluorescent staining of the V chromosome. Of particular value are undescended testes and inguinal hernia – the most common anomalies seen in children with hypospadias. Urine and plasma steroid levels are evaluated in combination with stimulation tests, though caution must be exercised in interpreting the values in the newborn. In addition to these basic investigations, radiographic procedures including genitography and voiding cystourethrography are very useful for excluding the presence of remnants of the müllerian ducts, such as a cervix or uterus. Sonography of the pelvis and endoscopic evaluation of the sinus urogenitalis, a blind vaginal pouch, and the urethra complete the diagnostic work-up. Only in those few patients with XY karyotype and presence of a cervix it is necessary to carry out exploratory laparotomy and gonadal biopsy. Another criterion for obtaining information is the measurement of testosterone metabolism and androgen binding in cultured fibroblasts (Bartsch et al. 1986).

Based on the endocrinological aspects of somatic differentiation and the mechanism of androgen action, several causative factors can be assumed to lead to ambiguity of the external genitalia (Brown et al. 1981; Goldstein and Wilson 1972; Imperato-McGinley et al. 1974; Keenan et al. 1974; Tunn et al. 1981; Wilson and MacDonald 1978): (a) inadequate biosynthesis of testosterone, (b) inadequate synthesis of dihydrotestosterone (5α-reductase deficiency), (c) androgen-binding deficiency, and (d) absence of müllerian duct regression.

With defective testosterone biosynthesis, patients show low plasma testosterone and dihydrotestosterone levels and, as a consequence, high gonadotropin secretion and negative human chorionic gonadotropin (HCG) stimulation. Five enzymatic defects resulting in ambiguity of the external genitalia during embryogenesis have been described. As plasma testosterone is very low during the neonatal period, measurement before and after stimulation with HCG is advisable to check the capacity for testosterone synthesis. Normally, the results after application of HCG show elevated plasma testosterone. A 5α-reductase deficiency demonstrates testosterone within normal limits, while dihydrotestosterone is markedly decreased. The serum levels for estradiol-17β are normal, whereas the luteinizing hormone (LH) values range from normal to elevated. HCG stimulation demonstrates a good response of the Leydig cells, with elevated testosterone. The fibroblast strains derived from genital tissue reveal a complete loss or diminution of 5α-reductase enzyme. The binding of 5α-dihydrotestosterone to the androgen receptor is normal.

In androgen-binding deficiency, individuals have been found to have either a decreased amount of an apparently normal androgen receptor or a qualitatively abnormal receptor. High testosterone, estradiol-17β, and LH levels are detected. In newborn babies, gonadal stimulation with HCG causes a significant rise in serum testosterone. Cultured fibroblasts from genital skin appear to have normal 5α-reductase activity.

Medical Treatment of Patients with Micropenis

Normal embryogenesis results in a properly formed penis at the 14th week of gestation. During the last two trimesters of pregnancy, the size of the normal penis increases considerably – about tenfold by the time of birth. In this period of pregnancy, androgen secretion is an important factor in promoting growth of the penis.

Perineoscrotal hypospadias is often associated with a microphallus, presenting a difficult surgical challenge, with a higher risk of complications and unsatisfactory results (Allen 1978; Kogan and Williams 1977; Swyer 1955; Walsh et al.

Table 1. Success rate after administration of human chorionic gonadotropins to patients with hypogonadotropic hypogonadism

Reference[a]	Patients (n)	Success rate
Allen (1978)	3	+[b]
Klugo and Cerny (1978) (1 000 E every 7 days for 3 weeks)	5	−[c] (14%)
Kogan and Williams (1977) (1 000 E every 7 days for 6 weeks)	2	1+, 1−
Bartsch et al. (1982) (1 500 E every 7 days for 4 weeks)	4	+

[a] Dose given in parentheses if known.
[b] Response to therapy.
[c] No response.

1978; Wilson and MacDonald 1978). Only recently has this problem begun to receive the attention it deserves. Preoperative enlargement should be performed before starting surgical intervention in a child with hypospadias and a small phallus. Besides the traditional treatment with testosterone either as an injection or as cream applied locally, various therapeutic approaches have been discussed for aberrant development of the penis and corresponding hormonal regulation. Of importance is the fact that good improvements – with effective phallic growth after hormonal stimulation – can only be achieved in endocrinological disorders. Emphasis should be placed on early therapy during childhood to attain the best response. Application of androgens has no effect in either postpubertal or adult patients.

Administration of gonadotropins produces genital growth and has proven to be an effective method to correct defective virilization and fertility in patients with hypogonadotropic hypogonadism (Table 1). Apart from HCG or combined HCG-human menopausal gonadotropin (HMG) therapy, testosterone is used for hormonal stimulation. The mechanism of growth is considered to be a local effect or systemic response. Smith treated 20 patients with testosterone injections according to the schedule outlined by Guthrie et al. some years before (Guthrie et al. 1973). Both reported a good increase in penis length, but results of long-term follow-up are lacking. Kogan and Williams (1977) noted the presence of a palpable testis to be a clinically useful diagnostic factor indicating testosterone treatment. Nevertheless, even if the patient primarily responds well to testosterone application, normal growth does not continue after artificial stimulation has been stopped.

Testosterone applied topically in various concentrations has been used effectively by several clinicians (Table 2): Darby et al. (1974), Immergut et al. (1971) and Allen (1978) administered the hormone in a low dose cream, whereas Klugo and Cerny (1978) observed the best growth in prepubertal male subjects after having applied 10% testosterone cream topically for local absorption twice daily. The earlier this therapy is instituted, the greater the likelihood of an excellent response. Attention must be paid to possible side effects, such as premature production of pubarche or accelerated bone growth.

Table 2. Success rate after topical application of testosterone to patients with microphallus

Reference[a]	Patients (*n*)	Success rate
Darby et al. (1974) (2.5%)	3	–[b]
Immergut et al. (1971) (5%)	1	+[c]
Allen (1978) (1%, 3%)	3	1+, 2–
Klugo and Cerny (1978) (10%)	5	+(60%)

[a] Concentration of testosterone given in parentheses.
[b] No response to therapy
[c] no response.

Dihydrotestosterone is responsible for the development and virilization of the external genitalia and male urethra. Diffusion of dihydrotestosterone in adults after application of 12.5 mg/day was pharmacologically tested, and serum levels four times as high as those in untreated persons were obtained. These findings justify the use of 5α-dihydrotestosterone to induce growth of the phallus. After a 4-week course of therapy in 45 patients with hypospadias and 5 with epispadias, good results were achieved with no significant complications. But again, discontinuation of treatment leads to a 50% decrease of penile growth (Bartsch et al. 1982, 1986; Montford and Lucas 1982).

Gender Assignment

The decision whether affected newborn males should be raised as males or females depends on the anatomic defect and on the feasibility of male or female reconstructive surgery. The decision is also influenced by the age of the patient at presentation – assignment should be made as early as possible, involving the parents in the decision-making process. In the newborn, an assessment must be made, taking into account the realities of future gender identity, the utility of the organ, sexual function, and any associated psychologic problems. Later on in childhood (normal psychosexual identity being well differentiated at the age of 2 years), and especially after the beginning of puberty, the clinician is often faced with a major dilemma (Crawford et al. 1970; Federmann 1967; Griffin/Wilson 1986; Lubs et al. 1959; Morris 1953). Besides the problems associated with operative correction, the psychosexual development and social environment have to be taken into consideration in every individual case. Since it is possible to induce penile growth by early testosterone therapy in patients with inadequate biosynthesis of testosterone, and since these patients identify themselves as males, reconstructive surgery should be performed in the male direction following testosterone therapy. Patients with severe anatomic defects of the phenotypical appearance should be raised as females, and surgical procedures (correction of the external genitalia and castration) should be started promptly to avoid virilization. The application of suitable estrogen is necessary at the time of expected puberty to promote development of normal female secondary sex characteristics. Therapy with glucocorticoids – and, in some instances, mineralocorticoids – is indicated in a combined defect of testosterone and corticoid biosynthesis.

Patients with 5α-reductase deficiency should be treated topically or systemically with 5α-dihydrotestosterone to stimulate penile growth. Since patients take on a male identity, reconstructive surgery should be performed in the male direction. Sometimes, one cannot make a diagnosis and decision for further treatment of patients raised as females before the menarche is missed and normal female breast development is observed; gonadectomy should then be performed immediately and estrogen substitution started (Imperato-McGinley et al. 1974).

Patients with severe hypospadias who are resistant to androgens should undergo reconstructive surgery in the female direction and should be raised as females. This is clearly shown in a patient who was operated on for perineal hypospadias. Moreover, he may serve as a cautionary example of delayed gender assignment and bad diagnosis. At a recent work-up, the patient showed diminished androgen binding, normal 5α-reductase in fibroblast culture, and high levels of gonadotropins. On physical examination, he presented a micropenis and gynecomastia. As a child, this patient should have been treated with reconstruction in the female direction.

Therapy

Hypospadias surgery requires meticulous attention to detail, and a successful outcome reflects the experience and ability of the surgeon involved. Adequate reconstruction demands above all straightening of the shaft (orthoplasty) so that normal intercourse is possible. This must be followed by urethroplasty, extending the neourethra up to, or to a point near, the tip of the glans, so that semen can be deposited deep in the vagina. More than 200 different procedures for hypospadias repair are described in the literature, all aimed at improving the function of the penis as a sex and urinary organ, and, of course, at achieving a good cosmetic result, e.g., by rearrangement of the dorsal skin. To assure the success of all surgical procedures, certain rules and principles of plastic surgery must be observed: atraumatic handling of the tissue, use of noncrushing instruments, special suturing techniques, and proper wound dressing. Diversion of the urine from the operative site is of paramount importance.

If after early and proper investigation the decision is made to perform corrective surgery in the male direction, one- or multistage repair should be carried out, depending on the degree of hypospadias (Bartsch and Pauer 1981; Bartsch et al. 1986; Marberger 1968; Marberger and Marberger 1962; Marberger and Pauer 1981; Schmid 1961). In the management of posterior hypospadias, single-stage procedures – such as those proposed by Devine – carry a high risk of persistent ventral deviation, microphallus, and, therefore, poor results.

We prefer a staged approach. In the first session, the penis is straightened by dissecting the chorda meticulously off the penile shaft until normal corpus spongiosum is reached between the crura penis. The opening of the hypospadic urethra is excised and separated from the penoscrotal skin. Then, the resulting epithelial defect is covered with a rotated flap, and the urethral stump is reimplanted. Mobile skin flaps are provided by two asymmetrical halves of the veillike expanded dorsal prepuce. The neourethra is formed with hairless skin by means of a pri-

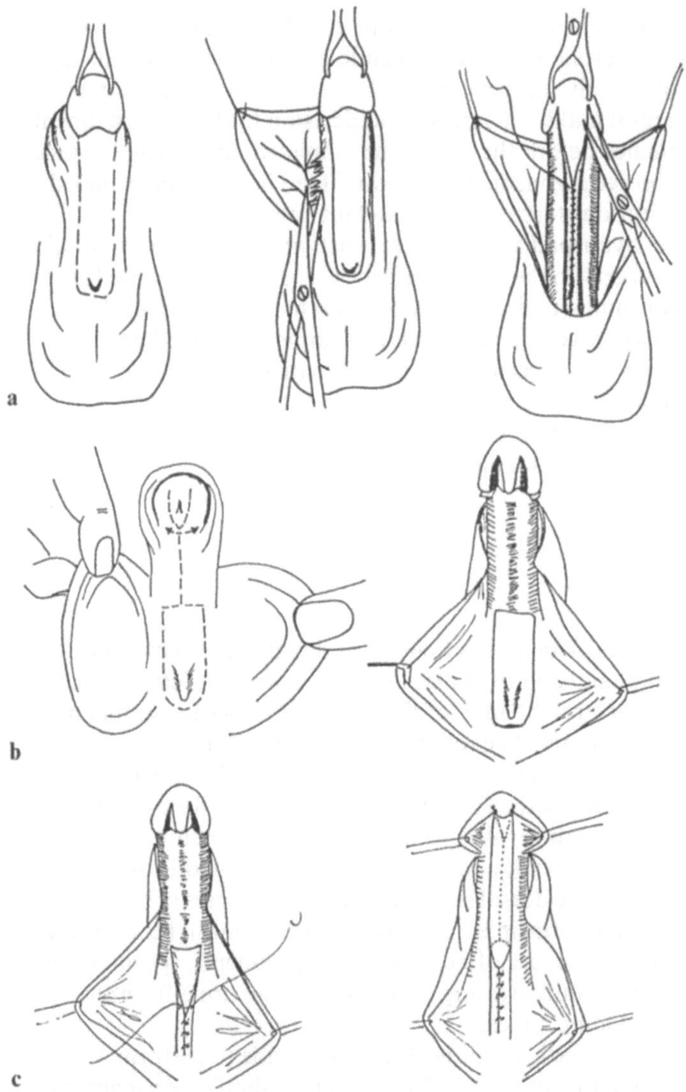

Fig. 3 a–c. Second stage of surgical correction of perineoscrotal hypospadias: construction of the urethra. (From Marberger 1968)

marily sutured tube in the second stage; the urethra is buried using wide mobilized penoscrotal skin flaps. Special attention is given to the development of a non-shrinking meatus (Figs. 3, 4).

Between 1952 and 1984, 96 patients with perineoscrotal meatus (77 scrotal, 19 perineal) and a bifid scrotum underwent surgical correction in our institution. In 8 patients, it was decided to perform feminization, including removal of the gonads and long-term substitutional hormone therapy, while 88 patients were treated using a staged approach as described above. Extended endocrine evaluaa 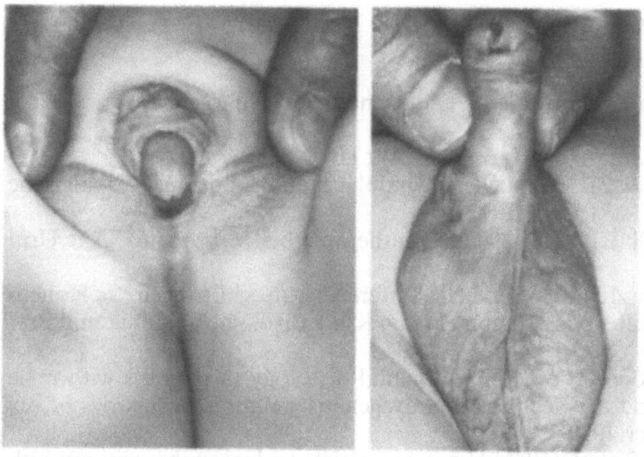 b

Fig. 4 a, b. One-stage correction of perineoscrotal hypospadias. (From Devine 1983)

tion to obtain a precise diagnosis – and, if necessary, preoperative androgen stimulation to effect growth of the phallus – has been carried out since 1980.

In 76 patients, correction after a two-stage procedure has been completed, and early and long-term results are available. The fistula rate was 6%, and in 8% of the patients, an anastomotic stricture or meatal stenosis was observed. In 14 patients, there was a poor cosmetic appearance but a good functional result.

A child with well-documented androgen receptor deficiency should, as early as possible, be raised as a female after undergoing feminizing genitoplasty (Goodwin 1981; Lattimer 1961; Mollard et al. 1981; Sotiropoulos et al. 1976; see also J.E. Altwein and J. Homoki, this volume). Clitoroplasty is performed in the 1st year of life by reducing the microphallus and forming a clitoris, being careful to spare the neurovascular bundle and to prepare a normal vestibulum and introitus vaginae. Vaginoplasty is carried out later, in a second step – especially in severe cases – in order to achieve good results. Sometimes, a neovagina (ileal or sigmoid) has to be constructed.

In patients with abnormalities of testosterone synthesis or 5α-reductase deficiency, the major criterion is the degree of masculinization of the external genitalia. Testosterone or 5α-dihydrotestosterone application is of great help in predicting what will occur at puberty, though in many cases, the patient will not be fertile. If one of the gonads is a streak or testicle – as in mixed gonadal dysgenesis – corrective surgery is carried out in the female direction. All patients have a uterus and vagina, and since as many as one-fourth of these individuals may develop gonadal tumors, the gonads – streak or testicles – should be removed. In general, the development of the external genitalia is the main criterion, whereas considerations of fertility are always of secondary importance.

References

Allen TD (1978) Microphallus: clinical and endocrinological characteristics. J Urol 119:750

Bartsch G, Pauer W (1981) Plastik nach Marberger. Akt Urol 5:38

Bartsch G, Schweikert HU (1982) Männlicher Pseudohermaphroditismus: ätiologische und diagnostische Aspekte. Akt Urol 13:121

Bartsch G, Schweikert HU, Glatzl J (1982) Hormontherapie bei Mikropenis. Akt Urol 13:74

Bartsch G, Schweikert HU, Glatzl J (1986) Sexuelle Differenzierungsstörungen. In: Hohenfellner R, Thüroff JW, Schulte-Wissermann H (eds) Kinderurologie in Klinik und Praxis. Thieme, Stuttgart New York p 459

Bergada C, Cleveland WW, Jones HW (1962) Gonadal histology in patients with male pseudohermaphroditism and atypical gonadal dysgenesis: relation to theories of sex differentiation. Acta Endocr 40:493

Brown TR, Maes M, Rothwell S et al. (1981) Human complete androgen insensitivity with normal dihydrotestosterone binding capacity in cultured genital skin fibroblasts: evidence for a qualitative abnormality of the receptor. J Clin Endocr 55:61

Crawford JD, Adams RD, Kliman B et al. (1970) Syndromes of testicular feminization: an informal appraisal and review of the latest advances and insights, with special emphasis on pathogenesis, biochemical mechanism at work and psychosocial clinical problems. Clin Pediat 9:165

Darby CW, Vanderschueren-Lodeweyck M, Laurance BM (1974) Testosterone cream: use or abuse? Lancet II:598

Devine CH jr (1983) Chordee and hypospadias. In: Glenn J (ed) Urologic surgery. Lippincott, Philadelphia p 775

Federmann DD (1967) Abnormal sexual development. Saunders, Philadelphia 1976

Forest MG (1975) Pattern of plasma testosterone and Δ 4androstenedione in normal newborns: evidence for testicular activity at birth. J Clin Endocr 41:977

Fredrick W, Wilson JD (1986) Embryology of the genital tract. In: Walsh PC, Gittes RF, Perlmutter AD, Stamey TA (eds) Campbells urology. 5th ed. Saunders, Philadelphia p 1804

Goldstein JL, Wilson JD (1972) Studies on the pathogenesis of the pseudohermaphroditism in the mouse with testicular feminization. J Clin Invest 51:1647

Goodwin W (1981) Partial (segmental) amputation of the clitoris for female pseudohermaphroditism. Soc Pediatr Urol (Newsletter)

Griffin JE, Wilson JD (1986) Disorders of sexual differentiation. In: Walsh PC, Gittes RF, Perlmutter AD, Stamey TA (eds) Campbells urology, 5th ed. Saunders, Philadelphia, p 1819

Guthrie RD, Smith DW, Graham CB (1973) Testosterone treatment for micropenis during early childhood. J Pediat 83:274

Immergut M, Boldus R, Yanone E et al. (1971) The local application of testosterone cream to the prepuberal phallus. J Urol 105:905

Imperato-McGinley J, Guerrero L, Gautier T et al. (1974) Steroid 5α-reductase deficiency in man: an inherited form of male pseudohermaphroditism. Science 186:1213

Jost A (1953) Problems of fetal endocrinology: the gonadal and hypophyseal hormones. Recent Progr Hormone Res 8:379

Jost A (1972) A new look at the mechanism controlling sex differentiation in mammals. Johns Hopkins Med J 130:38

Keenan BS, Meyer WJ, Hadjian AJ et al. (1974) Syndrome of androgen insensitivity in man: absence of 5α-dihydrotestosterone binding protein in skin fibroblasts. J Clin Endocr 38:1143

Klugo CR, Cerny JC (1978) Response of micropenis to topical testosterone and gonadotropin. J Urol 119:667

Kogan StJ, Williams DI (1977) The micropenis syndrome: clinical observations and expectations for growth. J Urol 118:311

Lattimer JK (1961) Relocation and recession of the enlarged clitoris with preservation of the glans: an alternative to amputation. J Urol 86:113
Lubs HA, Vilar O, Bergenstal DM (1959) Familial male pseudohermaphroditism with labial testes and partial feminization: endocrine studies and genetic aspects. J Clin Endocr 19:1110
Marberger H (1968) Hypospadieoperation unter Verwendung von asymmetrischen Präputiallappen. Urologe 7:161
Marberger H, Marberger E (1962) Ein Beitrag zum Problem des Pseudohermaphroditismus. Urol Int 13:65
Marberger H, Pauer W (1981) Experience in hypospadias repair. Urol Clin North Am 8:403
Mollard P, Juskiewenski S, Sarkissian J (1981) Clitoroplasty in intersex: a new Technique. Brit J Urol 53:371
Montfort G, Lucas C (1982) 5α-Dihydrotestosterontherapie zur Wachstumsstimulation des Penis vor der Hypospadiekorrektur. Akt Urol 13:79
Morris JM (1953) The syndrome of testicular feminization in male pseudohermaphrodites. Amer J Obstet Gynec 65:1192
Nowakowski H, Lenz W (1961) Genetic aspects in male hypogonadism. Recent Progr Hormone Res 17:53
Schmid MA (1961) Plastische Korrektur des äußeren Genitales bei einem männlichen Scheinzwitter. Arch klin Chir 298:977
Siiteri PK, Wilson JD (1974) Testosterone formation and metabolism during male sexual differentiation in the human embryo. J Clin Endocr 38:113
Simpson JL, New M, Peterson RE (1971) Pseudovaginal perineoscrotal hypospadias in sibs. Birth defects 7:140
Sotiropoulos A, Morishima A, Homsy Y, Lattimer JK (1976) Long-term assessment of genital reconstruction in female pseudohermaphrodites. J Urol 115:599
Swyer GIM (1955) Male pseudohermaphroditism: a hitherto undescribed form. Brit Med J 1955/II:709
Tunn UW, Weissbach L, Neumann F, Schweikert HU (1981) Hypospadie als Folge eines gestörten Androgenstoffwechsels und als Symptom der Intersexualität. Akt Urol 12:89
Walsh PC, Madden JD, Harrod MJ et al. (1974) Familial incomplete male pseudohermaphroditism, type 2: decreased dihydrotestosterone formation in pseudovaginal perineoscrotal hypospadias. New Engl J Med 291:944
Walsh PC, Wilson JD, Allen TD et al. (1978) Clinical and endocrinological evaluation of patients with congenital microphallus. J Urol 120:90
Wilson JD, MacDonald (1978) Male pseudohermaphroditism due to androgen resistance: testicular feminization and related syndromes. In: Stanbury JB, Wyngaarden JB, Frederickson DS (eds) The metabolic basis of inherited disease. McGraw-Hill, New York, p 894

Sexual Rehabilitation in Bladder Exstrophy

C. R. J. Woodhouse

The Academic Unit, The Institute of Urology, The Shaftesbury Hospital, Shaftesbury Avenue, London, WC2H8JE, UK

Introduction

Fifty years ago, exstrophy of the bladder was considered to be a largely fatal abnormality. At least half the patients died before the age of 10 years (Mayo and Hendricks 1926). Reconstructive surgery of the basic bladder condition has progressed so much that the patients can now live a normal life, and in the last 15 years have been able to expect to have a normally working bladder (Arap et al. 1980; Duckett and Caldemone 1984; Light and Scott 1984). Fortunately, there are very few associated abnormalities.

Urologists are faced with adolescent and adult patients who have grown up in normal society, gone to normal schools, taken normal jobs and developed the normal expectations of young people. The main problem is their conspicuously abnormal genitalia.

The policy of the Institute of Urology and St Peter's Hospitals is to continue the care of children with urological problems in a specialised adolescent urology clinic. The patients are drawn mainly from the combined paediatric urology unit of the Institute and the Hospital for Sick Children, Great Ormond Street. Some patients are referred from other hospitals at home and abroad. The patients are never discharged from the adolescent clinic, no matter how old they get. There are just over 100 adult exstrophy patients in the series.

It is clear both from our own patients and from the experience of other groups that exstrophy patients grow up very well (Jeffs 1978; Lattimer et al. 1979a; Woodhouse et al. 1983). They are highly motivated and hard-working people, who make light of their problems. Their libido is high. It is a matter of priority to reconstruct the genitalia to allow normal intercourse to take place.

Women

The problems in the women are relatively simple: Because the bladder and anterior abdominal wall are effectively missing, the vagina and anus are displaced forwards (Fig. 1). Indeed, in some patients, even after successful bladder reconstruction, the introitus appears to be on the lower abdomen rather than in the perineum (Fig. 2). The introitus is usually narrow, and in most cases, the narrowed part is short and is easily opened by an episiotomy. Only six patients have required a formal vaginoplasty (Table 1). When vaginoplasty is necessary, the posterior wall is incised deeply, and the resulting defect is covered by rotating a flap from each of the labia minora.

Plastic Surgery in the Sexually Handicapped
Eds.: W. Eicher/Kubli/Herms

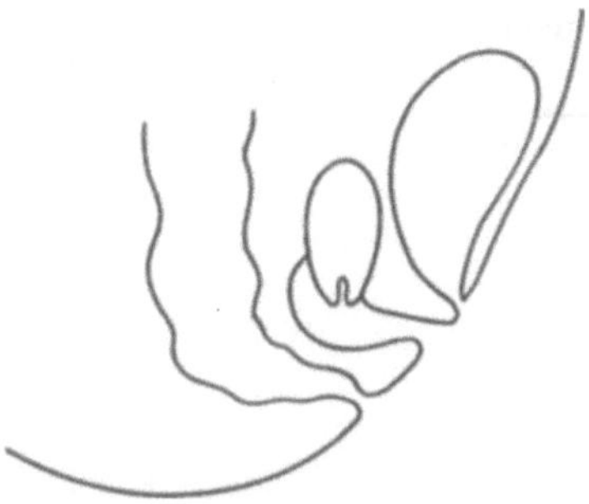

Fig. 1. Sagittal section of a female exstrophy patient, showing the relative positions of the pelvic organs. From *left* to *right*: rectum and anus, vagina and uterus, and bladder

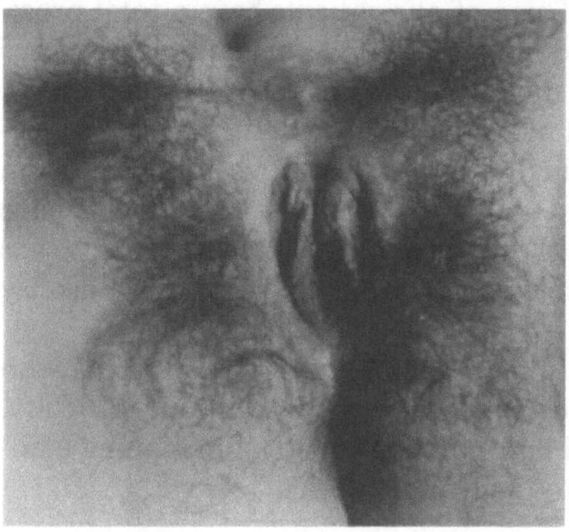

Fig. 2. The vulva in exstrophy. Note the anterior displacement of the structures compared to normal. The pubic hair is on either side of the vulva and is deficient in the midline over the mons due to the distribution of skin at the time of original bladder closure

Table 1. Vaginal surgery performed in 23 patients with bladder exstrophy

Surgery	Patients (*n*)
Episiotomy	6
Vaginoplasty	6
None (normal SI[a])	6
None (no SI or no information)	5

[a] Sexual intercourse.

The vagina runs directly posteriorly, so that when the patient is standing, the vagina is almost parallel with the floor; it is also rather shorter than usual. This arrangement does not interfere with intercourse, as Table 2 shows. The cervix enters the superior wall of the vagina and is very close to the introitus; this must contribute to the ease with which the girls get pregnant. It is essential to explain to the patients at an early stage that fertility is normal. Some girls have thought that they were so abnormal that conception was impossible. Of the 15 pregnancies in our patients, 2 have occurred because of this view, one of the girls having an intact hymen at the time of conception.

Table 2. Sexual function in 23 female patients with bladder exstrophy

Function	Patients (*n*)
Normal	14
Difficult	0
None	6
No information	3

The defective pelvic floor and poor uterine supports make prolapse common; it is a considerable problem to correct. Three of our patients have a total procidentia; one of these women has never had intercourse or a pregnancy. The uterus should not be removed, as it is the only solid organ in the pelvis that could possibly hold up the pelvic floor. The simplest procedure is to suture the lower segment of the uterus to the anterior abdominal wall with silk. If this fails, some form of sling should be put around the uterus: abdominal wall fascia or gracilis have been used. It must be said, however, that the management of uterine prolapse has presented great difficulty for the gynaecologists (Dewhurst et al. 1980; Blakeley and Mills 1981).

Eight women have had 15 children and 1 termination. Three patients who have urinary diversions were delivered of children vaginally without difficulty. Caesarean sections have been performed in five patients with a functioning bladder, which is safer than risking damage to the bladder outlet.

Men

Anatomy of the Exstrophy Pelvis

The problems for the men are much more troublesome. The penis is short and broad (Fig. 3), the shortness being due to deficiency in the length of the corpora and not to the split symphysis (Woodhouse and Kellett 1984). Cavernosograms

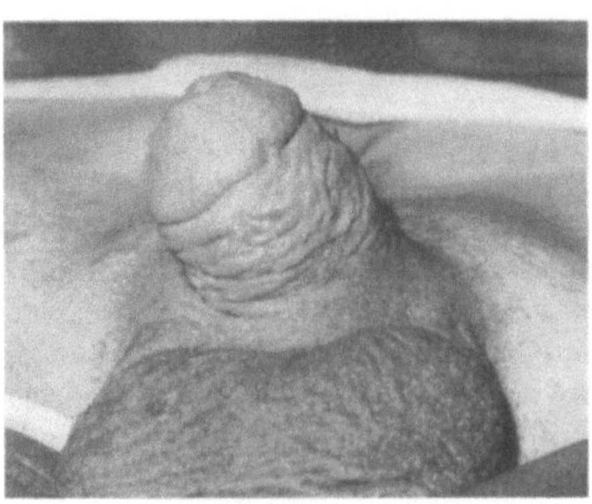

Fig. 3. Exstrophy penis in flaccid state

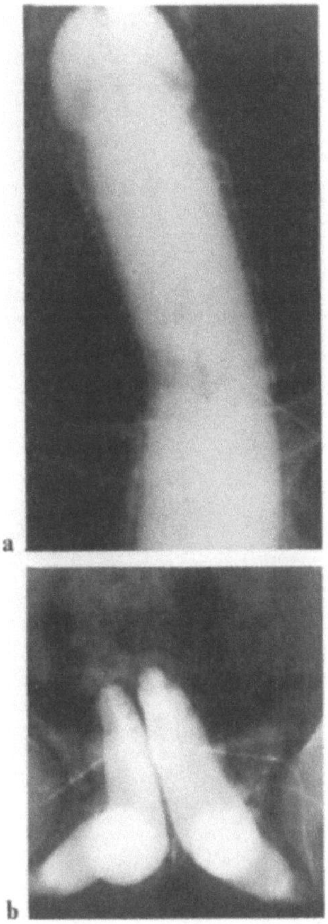

Fig. 4 a, b. Cavernosograms of **a** a normal penis and **b** an exstrophy penis

and computerised tomography (CT) scans demonstrate this quite clearly (Fig. 4, 5). When seen in the flaccid state, the penis certainly does not 'dangle'. Its shortness is emphasised by the normal size of the scrotum and the recession of the lower abdominal wall. Except in the rare cases where the penis has become buried in the scrotum due to previous surgery, no operation will make the exstrophy penis significantly longer. Johnston has shown that surgical apposition of the pubis does not lead to any penile lenghtening (1974).

The suggestion that the corpora could be completely detached from the inferior pubic rami and pulled forward has not stood the test of time (Kelley and Eraklis 1971): the work has never been followed up or repeated. It is certainly a theoretically dangerous procedure because of the risk of devascularising the corpora.

The orientation of the inferior pubic rami and the attachments of the deep parts of the corpora are unlike those of normal men. We have examined the cavernosograms of 16 adult exstrophies (Woodhouse and Kellett 1984). The pelvis is rotated caudally so that the inferior pubic rami are parallel with the floor when

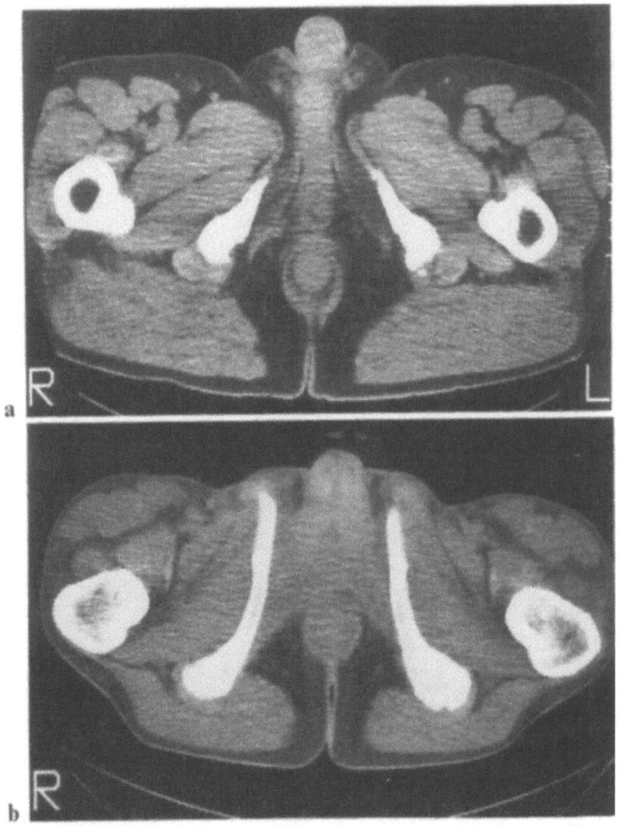

Fig. 5 a and b. Computerised tomograms at approximately the same level, showing sections through the lower pelvis of **a** a normal man and **b** an exstrophy patient. Note how short the deep parts of the corpora are in the exstrophy patient, especially from the anterior end of the inferior pubic ramus to the surface

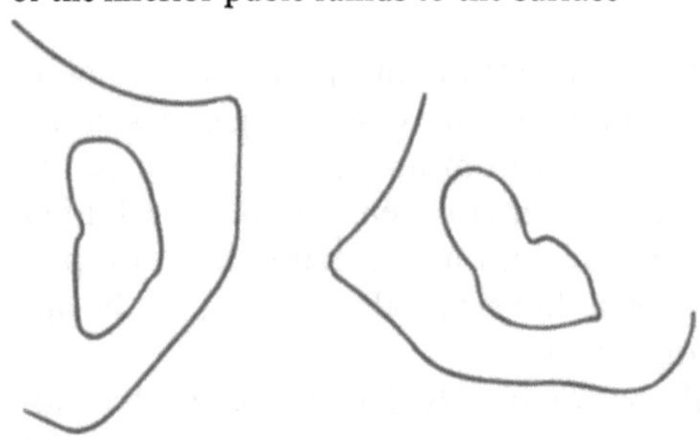

Fig. 6. Pelvic orientation in a normal man (*left*) and in an exstrophy patient (*right*)

the patient is standing (Fig. 6). Thus, no dissection posterior to the junction with the pubic body will give any lengthening.

If a young man with exstrophy has a short penis that is otherwise all rigt, there is nothing that can be done. Recent publications suggest that modern techniques of reconstruction lead to just this situation – a short but normal penis (Mesrobian et al. 1986). Thus, the management in adolescence consists of helping the boys to adjust to their abnormality. However, our experience with patients who are now young adults is that nearly all boys with exstrophy have an erectile deformity. In many, it is so severe that conventional sexual intercourse is impossible.

Erectile Deformities

We have identified three main types of erectile deformity (Woodhouse and Kellett 1984). The first two are uncommon and probably iatrogenic: they may arise through damage to one or both corpora during surgery in infancy.

Unilateral Rudimentary Corpus

If one corpus is damaged, it fails to fill properly on erection. It then acts as a bowstring on its fellow, so that the erection is pulled over to one side (Fig. 7). We have

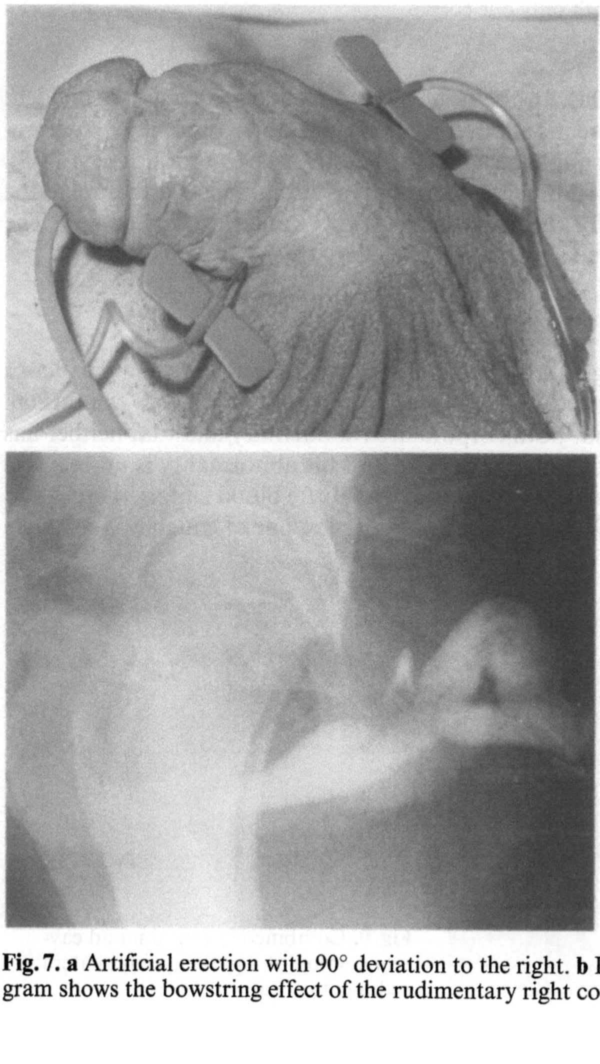

a

b

Fig. 7. a Artificial erection with 90° deviation to the right. **b** Lateral view of the cavernosogram shows the bowstring effect of the rudimentary right corpus

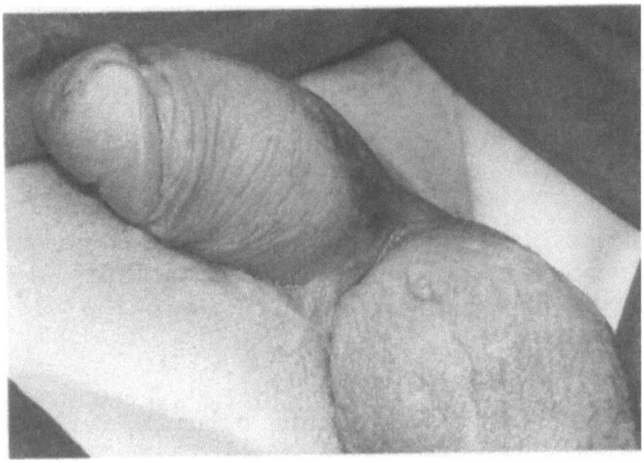

Fig. 8. Artificial erection after the division of the rudimentary corpus shown in Fig. 7. Note how unstable the erection is with only one corpus

only seen three cases like this. In the first, the rudimentary corpus was divided. This resulted in a straight erection, but it was very unstable: a proper erection requires the two corpora to support each other like the gables of a house (Fig. 8). For the second patient, the rudimentary corpus was straightened with dura in the way that will be described for the common deformity , and this worked well. The third patient has not come to surgery yet.

Bilateral Rudimentary Corpus

If both corpora are damaged, little erection occurs. Externally, the penis looks reasonable, though it is placed rather higher on the abdominal wall than usual. A cavernosogram shows that both corpora are rudimentary and that neither has any contact with the inferior pubic rami (Fig. 9). This abnormality is untreatable at present: penile surgery is likely to damage what little blood supply there is and thus abolish any erection. We have seen five examples, one of which was so severe

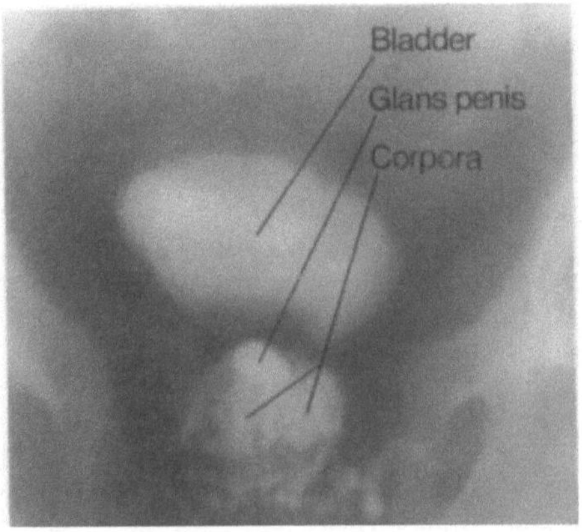

Fig. 9. Combined cystogram and cavernosogram of a patient with bilateral rudimentary corpora

that the patient had no visible penis at all, and only one of the patients has intercourse. The latter patient fractured his corpus during vigorous penetration, and it failed to heal spontaneously after 4 weeks. After localised surgical repair, he was impotent for several months but is now back to normal.

Dorsal Chordee

The most important erectile deformity is dorsal chordee. It seems likely that this is a normal component of the exstrophy complex, and it is seen in some degree in almost all adults with repaired exstrophy. It was seen in both patients who, for reasons best known to their mothers, had no treatment of any kind for their exstrophy until they were past 30 years old. It is seen in some degree in all patients with split symphysis epispadias who have had no penile surgery.

On erection, the penis is tightly curved and almost digs into the anterior abdominal wall (Fig. 10). The chordee is commonly so tight that normal vaginal penetration is impossible. Many patients are able to have a form of intercourse with the girl sitting astride (Fig. 11). Those who find satisfaction do not wish to

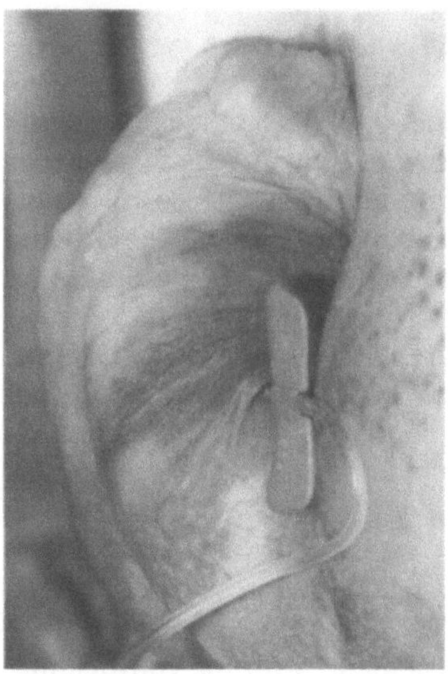

Fig. 10. Artificial erection showing the tight dorsal chordee that is the commonest erectile deformity in exstrophy

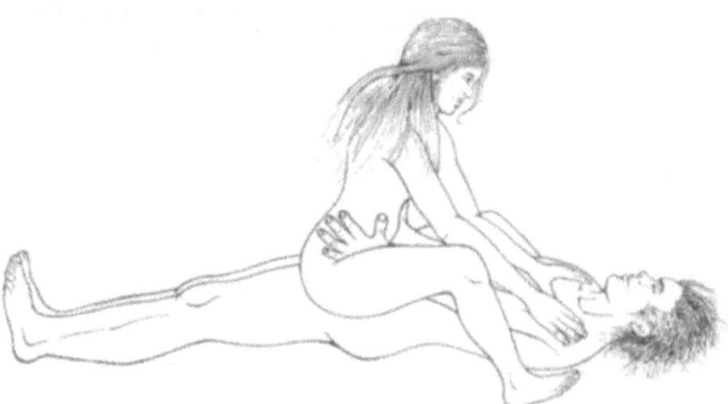

Fig. 11. A position adopted for intercourse when the dorsal chordee is uncorrected

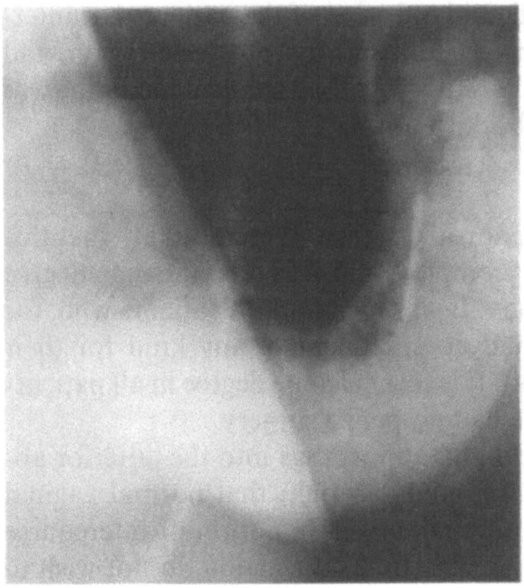

Fig. 12. Lateral view of a cavernosogram showing dorsal chordee

have a surgical correction. Many exstrophy patients have to use a syringe to inseminate their partners.

It might be thought that this deformity was due to the scar tissue around the dorsally placed urethra. Some authorities report that clearance of the scar and detachment of the urethra correct the chordee (Spehr and Melchior 1985). We have only found this to be so in 1 of 32 patients operated on. Although the original problem may have been a congenitally short urethral plate, by adulthood the basic problem is intrinsic curvature of the corpora (Fig. 12).

This type of erectile chordee is correctable. Careful selection of patients is important: it is preferable to wait until penile growth is complete at the end of puberty, and also until the boy has developed emotionally so that he understands the purpose of the operation. It is not satisfactory to embark on a programme of cosmetic operations if the patient cannot see anything wrong with the existing situation. If he has an understanding partner and has tried to have intercourse, it is a help, but I certainly would not wait until repeated failures have damaged the patient's ego.

In the early cases, a cavernosogram was always made, with the contrast medium being infused under a pressure of 300 mm Hg, to assess the nature of the problem before surgery (Hertzberg et al. 1981). This now seems unnecessary, if two good corpora are palpable in the perineum and there is no lateral deviation on erection.

Several methods of correcting the deformities of the exstrophy penis have been described (Johnston 1974; Hendren 1979; Koff and Eakins 1984; Woodhouse 1986). My approach includes some elements of most of these methods but relies mainly on the implantation of a patch of lyophilised human dura into the corpora.

The details of the operation will be found elsewhere (Woodhouse 1986). The principle is to expose the dorsal aspect of the corpora: clear all the scar tissue and then see what progress has been made by means of an artificial erection. It is

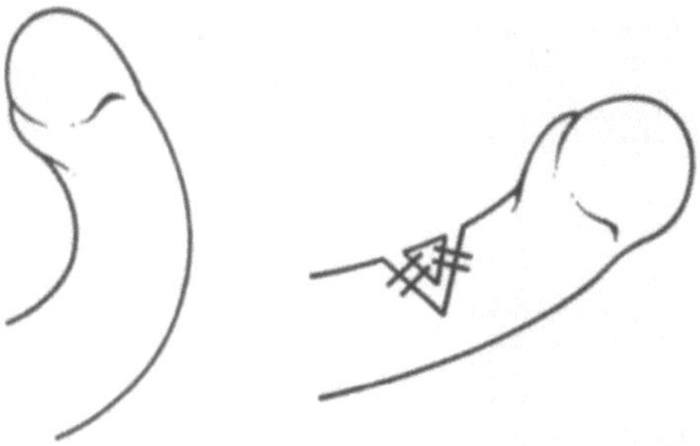

Fig. 13. The principle of chordee correction: incision of the concave aspect and insertion of an ellipse of lyophilised human dura

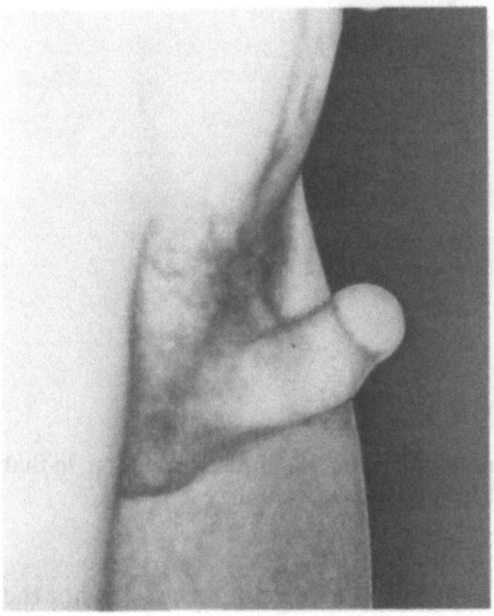

Fig. 14. Natural erection showing a good result of chordee correction by dural inlay. (Same patient as in Fig. 10)

usually necessary to divide the urethra and transpose it ventrally. Assuming that the penis is still not straight, the point of maximum curvature is incised, and the concave aspect is lengthened by the insertion of an ellipse of lyophilised human dura (Fig. 13). In closing the wound, skin flaps over the pubis are rotated to give a more natural distribution of pubic hair.

This is a long and tedious operation with a good deal of blood loss. The advantage of going to this amount of trouble to lenghten the concave curve is that the penis ends up slightly longer. A conventional Nesbitt's procedure, which shortens the convex curve, results in slight shortening. The disadvantage is that a second operation is necessary to reconstruct the urethra. Theoretically, the urethroplasty could be done at the first operation; however, I have not been keen to implant a foreign material such as dura and do a free graft of skin at the same time. On the rare occasions when there is enough skin to do a pedicled urethroplasty, a single stage is reasonable.

I have now performed 30 dural phalloplasties, of which 20 are assessable. Of these patients, 12 have had an excellent result on the first occasion, and 3 only after a revision (Fig. 14). Three patients have had a moderate result, in that there

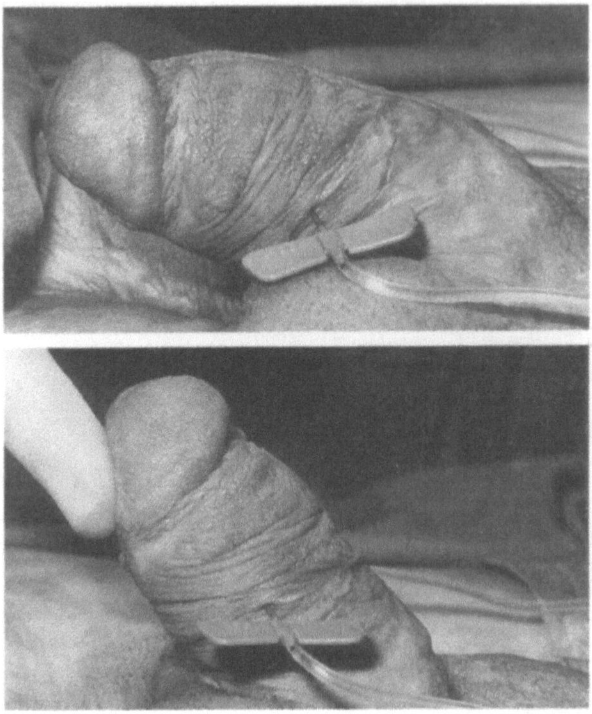

a

b

Fig. 15 a and b. Artificial erection showing a moderate result of chordee correction, in that there is less curvature and more flexibility but incomplete correction

is less curvature and more flexibility, even though the angle of erection is not the 40°–45° that I would like to achieve (Fig. 15). In two patients, the situation has not been improved.

All those in whom there was an improvement and who have had an appropriate opportunity have since been able to achieve limited vaginal penetration, the limitation being the overall penile length. I have not made a formal assessment of the quality of intercourse that the patient and his partner have, but I recognise that this is a very critical aspect and that casual opinions, especially from the operating surgeon, are valueless. A psychiatrist has just joined our team, and it is hoped that he will be able to report on this aspect before too long.

Sexual Function

With or without surgical correction, these boys appear to have a normal libido. It is our impression that they have fewer casual sexual partners than would be expected, and only one admits to being promiscuous. They appear to form very stable relationships with normal partners and have a normal life. Of the 43 patients for whom full information is available, 33 have been married or lived with a partner. Only one patient is known to be homosexual, and he is one of the three who have gone into the priesthood, possibly to avoid sexual responsibilities. One boy has doubts about his sexual identity and is an epispadiac rather than a true exstrophy patient: he may come to gender reassignment eventually. An unknown number of patients of all ages have not had any sexual contact, and for many of them the combination of abnormal genitalia and an external urinary diversion seems to be too overwhelming. Much of the operating time at present is taken up in the construction of internal continent diversions (Cumming et al. 1987).

Six men have initiated one or two pregnancies, from which there have been four children, and a further six are known to be infertile. These figures are broadly in line with those reported elsewhere (Lattimer et al. 1979 b). The main cause of infertility appears to be repeated prostatic and bladder infections. Thus, ironically, the boys who underwent early urinary diversion have the best record for fertility.

All the 19 offspring from our patients have been normal. From a postal survey of clinics all over the world, it has been reported that 1 in 70 offspring has exstrophy or epispadias (Shapiro et al. 1984); this figure must represent the worst that can be expected.

Conclusion

The exstrophy patient is born with an unpleasant but localised abnormality of the bladder and genitalia. Functional reconstruction of the bladder is now the norm. The children grow up to be very admirable members of society. If their genital abnormalities are not correct by surgery in infancy, these patients deserve very careful help and reconstruction in early adult life.

References

Arap S, Giron AM, Menzies de Goes G (1980) Initial results of the complete reconstruction of bladder exstrophy. Urol Clin North Am 7:477–491

Blakely CR, Mills WG (1981) The obstetric and gynaecological complications of bladder exstrophy and epispadias. Br J Obstet Gynaecol 88:167–173

Cumming J, Worth PHL, Woodhouse (1987) The choice of suprapubic continent catheterisable stoma. Br J Urol 60:227–230

Dewhurst J, Topliss PH, Shepherd JH (1980) Ivalon sponge hysteropexy for genital prolapse in patients with bladder exstrophy. Br J Obstet Gynaecol 87:67–69

Duckett JW, Caldemone AA (1984) Bladder exstrophy. AUA Update Series, lesson 13, vol 3, Houston, Texas

Hendren WH (1979) Penile lenghtening after previous repair of epispadias. J Urol 121:527–534

Herzberg Z, Kellett MJ, Morgan RJ, Pryor JP (1981) Method, indications and results of corpus cavernosography. Br J Urol 53:641–644

Jeffs RD (1978) Exstrophy and cloacal exstrophy. Urol Clin North Am 5:127–140

Johnston JH (1974) Lengthening of the congenital or acquired short penis. Br J Urol 46:685–687

Kelley JH, Eraklis AJ (1971) A procedure for lengthening the phallus in boys with exstrophy of the bladder. J Pediatr Surg 6:645–649

Koff SA, Eakins M (1984) The treatment of penile chordee using corporeal rotation. J Urol 131:931–932

Lattimer JK, Hensle TW, Macfarlane MT, Beale L, Braun E, Eposito Y (1979a) The exstrophy support team: a new concept in the care of the exstrophy patient. J Urol 121:472–473
Lattimer JK, Macfarlane MT, Puchor PJ (1979b) Male exstrophy patients: a preliminary report on the reproductive capability. Trans Am Assoc Genitourin Surg 70:42–46
Light JK, Scott FB (1984) The artificial urinary sphincter in children. Br J Urol 56:54–57
Mayo CH, Hendricks WA (1926) Exstrophy of the bladder. Surg Gynecol Obstet 43:129–134
Mesrobian H-GJ, Kelalis PP, Kramer SA (1986) Long term follow-up of cosmetic appearance and genital function in boys with exstrophy: review of 53 patients. J Urol 136:256–258
Shapiro E, Lepor H, Jeffs RD (1984) The inheritance of the exstrophy-epispadias complex. J Urol 132:308–310
Spehr C, Melchior HJ (1985) Operative correction of the penis deformity in bladder exstrophy. 20th Congress of the International Society of Urology, June 1985, Vienna, Abstr 1008, p 320
Woodhouse CRJ, Ransley PG, Williams DI (1983) The patient with exstrophy in adult life. Br J Urol 55:632–635
Woodhouse CRJ, Kellett MJ (1984) Anatomy of the penis and its deformities in exstrophy and epispadias. J Urol 132:1122–1124
Woodhouse CRJ (1986) The management of erectile deformity in adults with exstrophy and epispadias. J Urol 135:932–935

Congenital and Acquired Penile Deviations: Assessment and Surgical Correction

D. Yachia

Department of Urology, Hillel Yaffe Memorial Hospital, Hadera, Israel

Penile curvatures are defined as angulation of the penis during erections. According to Nesbit, the first congenital penile deviation was found and treated by Young in 1932, but it was Nesbit himself who first described this entity in 1954, and he later performed the procedure that we are still using to correct the deviation surgically (Nesbit 1965).

Bowlike penile curvatures can be seen on many ancient sculptures (Fig. 1), Greek vases, or wall paintings in Pompeii. These mostly mild curvatures probably did not disturb the subjects who served as models; however, severe curvature causes not only sexual dysfunction but also severe psychological problems.

Anatomically, the penis has three major components – the paired corpora cavernosa and, lying ventrally the corpus spongiosum, which contains the urethra. The glans penis is the terminal part of the corpus spongiosum (Fig. 2). The corpora are composed of highly vascularized connective tissue surrounded by a layer of strong connective tissue called tunica albuginea (Fig. 3).

Penile deviations can be congenital or acquired. The congenital ones are caused by asymmetric development of one of the corporal bodies. In the acquired deviations, part of the tunica albuginea becomes shorter for various reasons, as in Peyronie's disease or scarring of the tunica caused by penile "fractures." The curvatures in these conditions are usually to the right or to the left (Fig. 4) or dor-

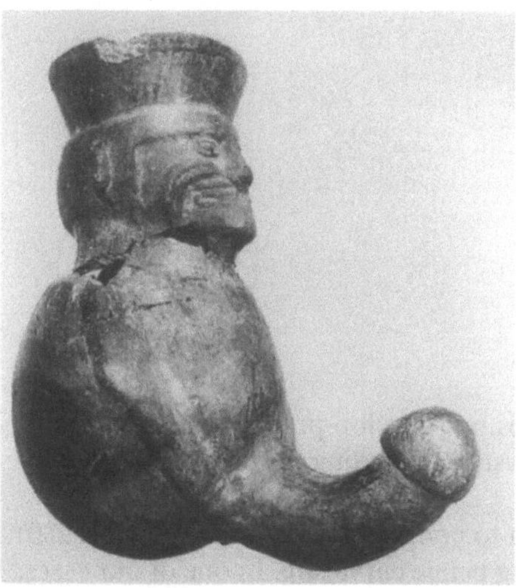

Fig. 1. Sculpture from Peru showing severe dorsal curvature

Plastic Surgery in the Sexually Handicapped
Eds.: W. Eicher/Kubli/Herms

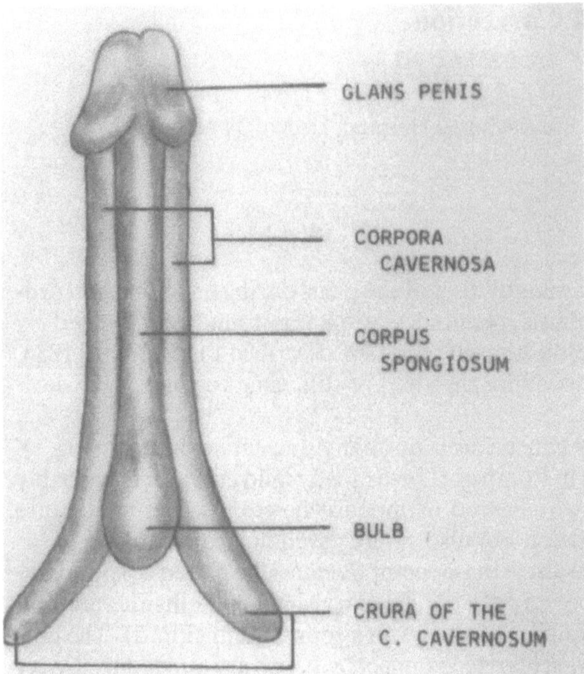

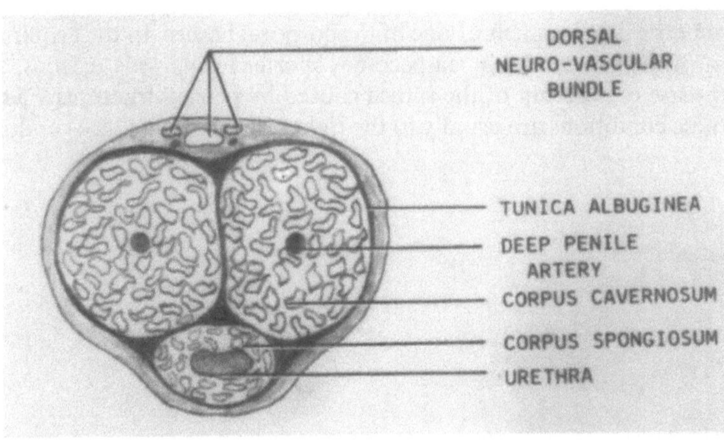

Fig. 3. Cross section of the penis

sal (Fig. 9). If the corpus spongiosum does not develop properly or becomes fibrotic for whatever reason, it acts as a bowstring, bending the penis markedly towards the urethra (Fig. 5).

There may be a familial predisposition to congenital curvature. Udall (1980) reported two cases of father and son having penile curvature. In one of our cases, the father of a 14-year-old boy told us about having a similar condition to that

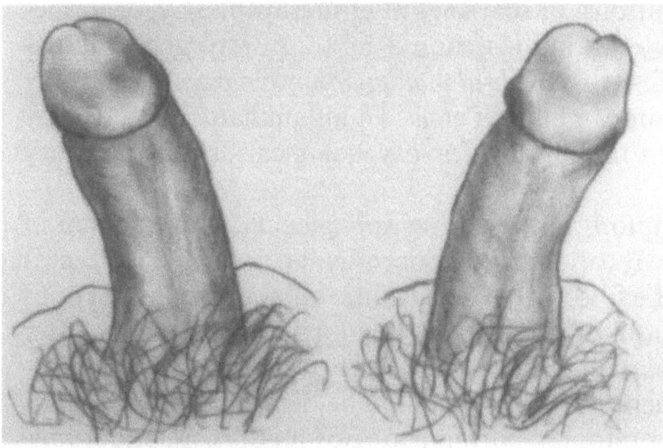

Fig. 4. Left and right lateral curvatures

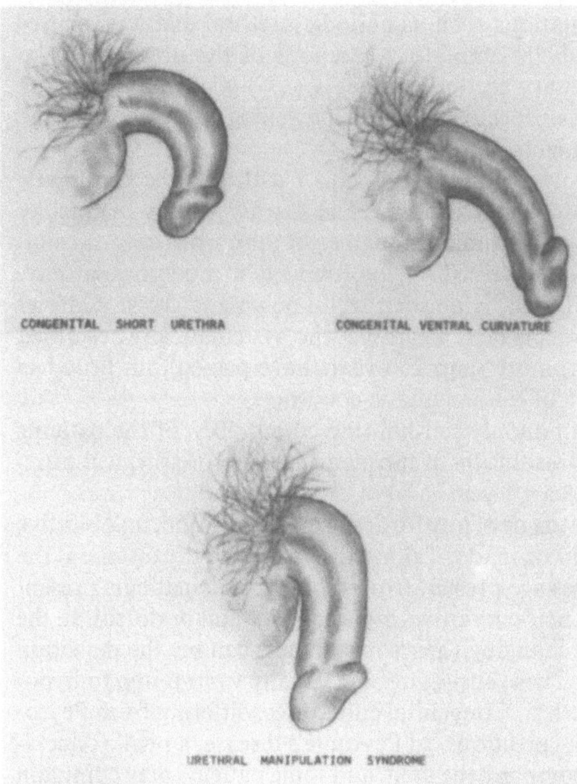

Fig. 5. Ventral curvature of various types

of his son, but with less curvature. The father did not have problems of penetration with any of his various partners; however, he asked for his son's penis to be corrected.

The acquired deviations are caused by chronic inflammatory diseases of the urethra leading to fibrosis of the corpus spongiosum. Such fibrosis can also be iatrogenic, being caused by transurethral surgical procedures, indwelling catheters, repeated urethral dilations, or scarrings after urethroplasties or unsuccessful chordee excisions. Penile deviations caused by transurethral manipulations were systematically described as *urethral manipulation syndrome* (UMS) by Kelâmi in 1984. Rarely, a patient can himself cause an inflammatory reaction by introducing foreign bodies into the urethra for psychological or masturbatory reasons.

Due to the fibrosis that develops in the corpus spongiosum, the deviation in UMS is always ventral (Fig. 5). It can only be noticed by the patient when the fibrosis is in the penile shaft: if the fibrosis develops at the bulbous urethra, it does not cause a deviation. When inquired about their erections, many patients, after repeated urethral manipulations, will report some degree of curvature and the disappearance of glans engorgement during erections. The disappearance of glans engorgement is a permanent symptom of corpus spongiosum fibrosis, and it cannot be treated surgically. In some UMS cases, the deviation straightens spontaneously when urethral manipulations such as periodic urethral dilations or frequent cystoscopies are stopped. Inflammatory reactions of the urethra can be minimized by avoiding unnecessary urethral trauma, i.e., by gentle handling; the use of small-caliber cystoscopes, resectoscopes, or indwelling catheters; and the use of pure silicone rubber catheters.

Peyronie's disease, also known as induratio penis plastica or the bent spike syndrome, is also an acquired benign process. The disease causes plaquelike thickenings of the elastic tissue of the tunica albuginea of the corpus cavernosum. Historically, this condition was described by the founder of modern anatomy, Andreas Vesalius, in 1538, and then by another well-known anatomist, Gabriel Fallopius, in 1561[1]. It was François de la Peyronie who systematically described the disease in 1743. Since then, more than 250 years have passed, but little has been learned about the etiology of this enigmatic condition.

Since the disease is most commonly self-limiting, about 50% of the patients show a complete, spontaneous resolution of the plaques; therefore surgical treatment should be delayed for at least 1 year.

Before proceeding with treatment of any form of penile deviation, an objective evaluation of the disease should be made. Taking the history of the disease is the first step. Congenital curvatures are present from birth, but the patients present after their 2nd decade of life. Their curvatures are usually lateral or dorsal. In the pediatric population, mothers changing their sons' diapers can see the deviation when the child's penis is erect. These curvatures are usually ventral due to hypospadias or congenital short urethra. Congenital curvatures, differing from Peyronie's disease, are painless during erections. In Peyronie's disease, a penile flaccidity distal to the plaque may accompany the pain, and some patients may complain of inability to initiate an erection. In some patients, the curvature is so severe that penetration becomes impossible. Inspection and palpation is the second step. Inspection of a flaccid penis usually does not reveal any abnormality, excepting hypospadic deformities. Plaques of Peyronie's disease, chordees, or fibrotic corpus spongiosum can be palpated easily.

---

[1] Andreas Vesalius (1514–1564): *Tabulae Anatomicae Sex* (1538), *De Humani Corporis Fabrica* (1543); Gabriel Fallopius (1523–1562): *Observationes Anatomicae* (1561)

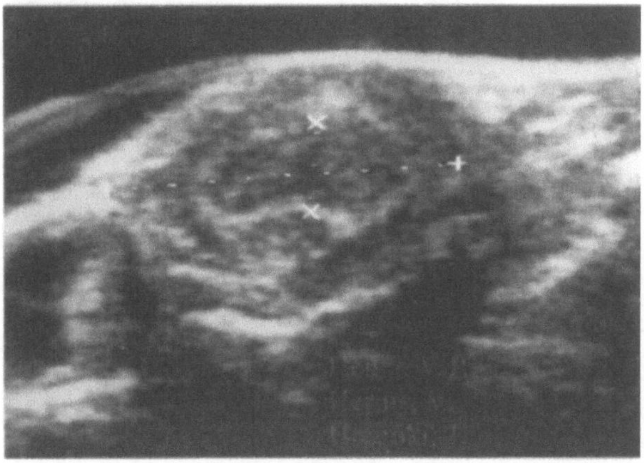

Fig. 6. Ultrasonogram of the penis (transverse section). Note the dorsal plaques (*x*)

Imaging of the penis is an important step in the evaluation of the problem. Sonography of the penis in Peyronie's disease helps to determine the extent of the plaques (Hamm et al. 1986). Normal corpora show a hyporeflective echo structure. The tunica albuginea is a thin, hyperreflective layer around the corpora. Plaques of Peyronie's disease are seen as hyperreflective thickenings in the tunica (Fig. 6). Detection of calcifications by their strong echogenicity and their typical posterior shadow facilitates the decision to undertake surgical treatment because calcified plaques do not disappear spontaneously. In UMS patients, fibrosis of the corpus spongiosum can be detected sonographically; however, the corpus spongiosum is not involved in Peyronie's disease. No changes of the tunica albuginea can be sonographically detected in congenital penile curvatures. The extent of the plaques can also be assessed by cavernosography. This is a small but invasive intervention that requires a small amount of irradiation to the genitals and has some morbidity. There have been reports of cases of erectile tissue fibrosis after injection of contrast material into the corpora.

Autophotography is the most objective method of evaluating penile curvatures. With these pictures, we can assess the degree of curvature, make a follow-up of progression or regression of the curvature, and compare results of surgical corrections. For autophotography we adopted the technique of Professor Kelâmi (1983, 1985). We either explain to the patient how to take the pictures or give him a copy of the instructions brochure explaining the following picture-taking positions:

1. The patient stands on a white floor or plain sheet (Fig. 7). With the penis fully erect, the picture is taken from above. This position documents lateral curvatures (Fig. 4).
2. The patient stands beside a white wall or door (Fig. 8). The camera is held with one hand at the level of the penis, with the other hand stabilizing the arm holding the camera; the picture is taken from the side. This position documents dorsal or ventral curvatures (Figs. 5, 9).
3. The patient holds the camera with both hands in front of the penis and takes the picture (Fig. 10). This position documents right or left curvatures (Fig. 11).

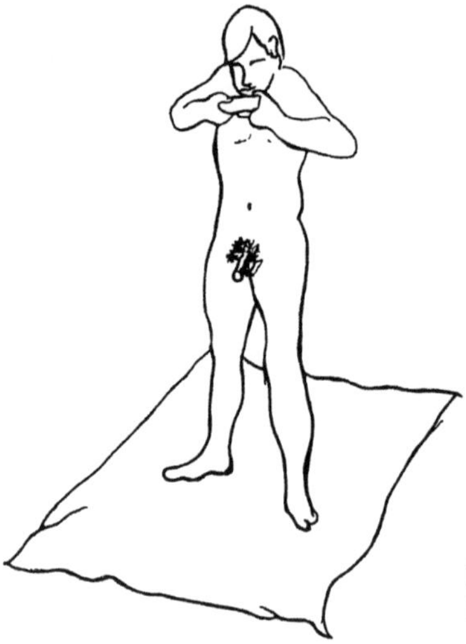

Fig. 7. Autophotography for documenting right or left lateral deviations

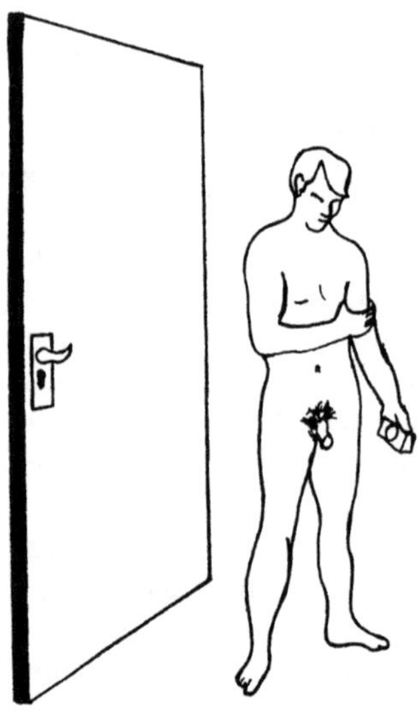

Fig. 8. Autophotography for documenting ventral or dorsal deviations

Curvatures of the penis are surgically curable lesions, but not every penile deviation needs to be corrected. Surgical correction is required when coital function is impaired; if the patient can penetrate without difficulty and both partners enjoy the sexual act, there is no need to try to straighten the penis. Difficulties in penetration depend not only on the severity of angulation but also on the anatomical condition of the sexual partner.

About 10% of patients with Peyronie's disease need surgical correction. The others either show a spontaneous resolution of the plaques or react favorably to the conservative but mostly empirical treatments given to them. Vitamin E tablets, the antifibroblastic agent Potaba (potassium *para*-aminobenzoate), orally

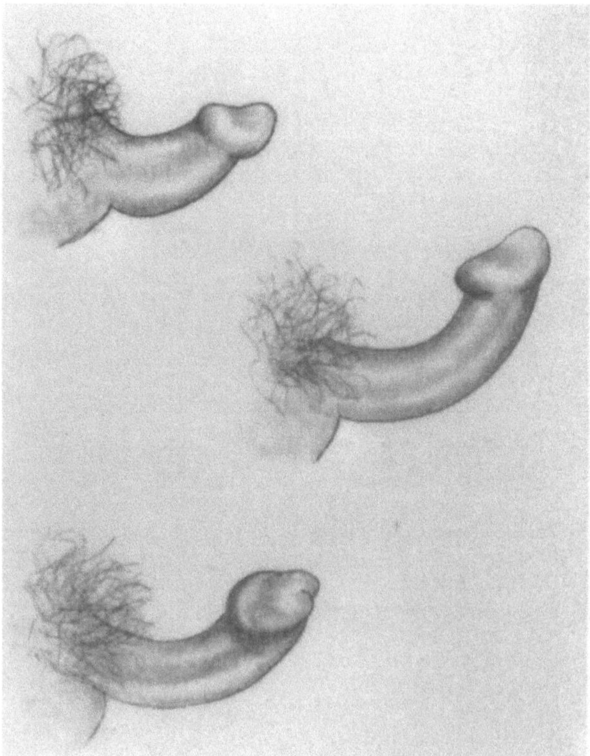

Fig. 9. Dorsal curvature of various types

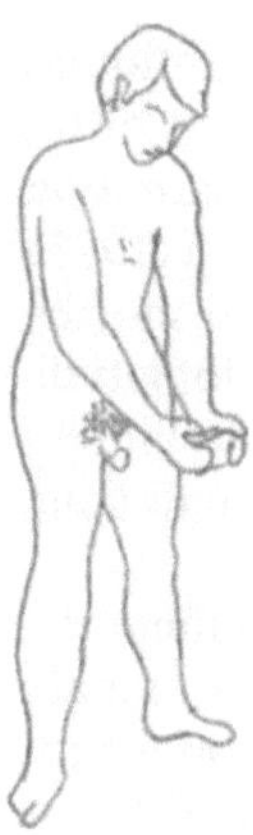

Fig. 10. Autophotography for documenting right or left deviations

administered corticosteroids, steroid injections into the plaques, local irradiations, or local ultrasound therapies may be tried. None of these treatments has been proved to be better than any other; however, they may be given until a regression occurs or a surgical correction is decided on. Penile curvatures can be corrected by three main surgical procedures, alone or in combination: (a) corporoplasty, (b) penile prosthesis implant, and (c) urethroplasty.

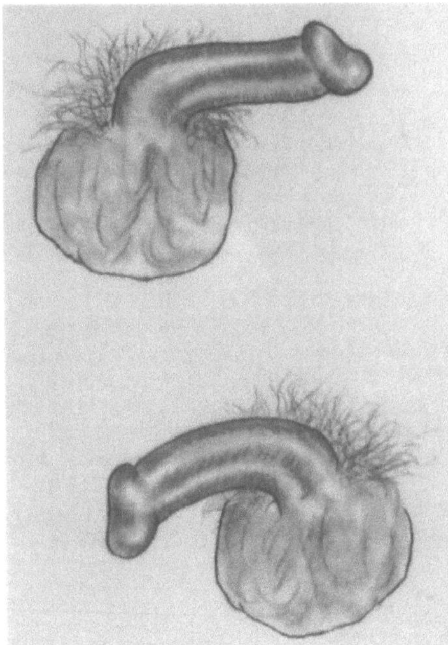

Fig. 11. Right and left lateral curvatures

Corporoplasty

Various corporoplasty techniques have been tried. Nesbit's procedure is an almost ideal primary repair for most penile curvatures, regardless of their etiology (Nesbit 1965). The principle of this procedure is to remove ellipsoid parts of the tunica albuginea from the longer corpus in order to make it equal in length to its counterpart. An alternative surgical technique proposed by Saalfield et al (1973), was based on the Heineke-Mikulicz principle: in order to lengthen the shorter, concave corpus, several transverse incisions are made and then closed longitudinally. This kind of repair causes a narrowing of the penis, whereas a Nesbit corporoplasty causes a shortening of the penis by 1–2 cm. None of our patients complained about this shortening.

Ebbehøj and Metz (1985), instead of removing parts of the tunica albuginea, proposed to make plications of the tunica by placing double-crossover, nonabsorbable stitches grasping deep into the tunica. Corporoplasties based on plaque excisions and patching of the gap with various materials – such as dermis (Devine and Horton 1974), tunica vaginalis (Das 1980), and lyophilized dura (Kelâmi 1980) – were designed for treatment of the curvatures caused by Peyronie's disease. These techniques were found to be far from satisfactory, as they resulted in a high incidence of impotence (Melman and Holland 1978; Pryor and Fitzpatrick 1979). It is unclear why grafting caused impotence.

Nowadays, the most widely used surgical technique for the correction of penile curvatures is Nesbit's procedure, in either its original form or its modifications.

This is a relatively simple operation, performed in one stage, and it requires only a short period of hospitalization. This technique has also been for the correction of childhood penile curvatures (Redman 1978); however, in children with a small penis I would prefer to delay the procedure until after puberty, when the penis reaches its adult size.

Surgical Technique

A Nesbit corporoplasty can be performed with the patient under spinal or general anesthesia. We do not use local anesthesia because infiltrating the penile skin with local anesthetics distorts the penis and makes it more difficult to retract the skin. A circular incision is made 0.5–1 cm under the corona, and the skin is retracted in the direction of the penile base. Occasionally, an infrapubic approach to the corpora cavernosa may be required. This approach is used when the cause of the curvature is UMS and the fibrosis of the corpus spongiosum is at the penoscrotal angle. The ellipsoid parts of the tunica are removed through the circular incision. After retracting the penile skin, a tourniquet is applied at the base of the penis, and an artificial erection is induced by injecting 50–100 ml saline through a 21-gauge butterfly canula inserted into one of the corpora cavernosa. Using Allis clamps, one or more "bites" are taken from the most convex part of the tunica albuginea, until the penis straightens. Lateral curvatures can be corrected by one or two excisions from the most convex point (Fig. 12). Dorsal curvatures are corrected by removing symmetrical ellipses from the ventral side of both corpora

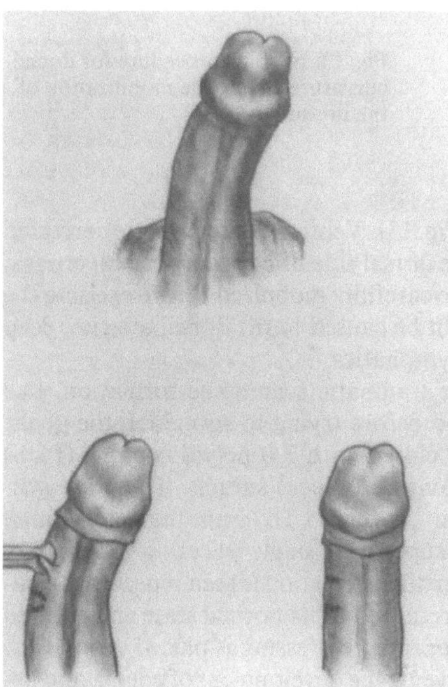

Fig. 12. Nesbit's procedure for lateral curvatures

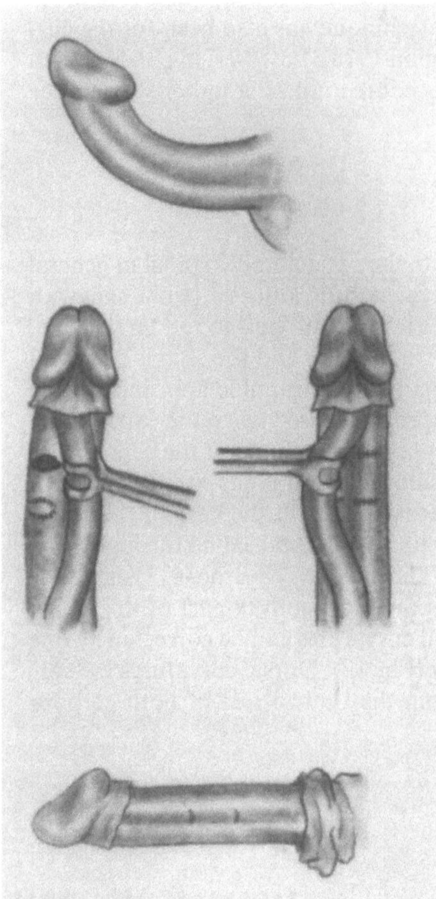

Fig. 13. Nesbit's procedure for dorsal curvatures. Note the mobilization of the urethra

cavernosa, after mobilizing the urethra (Fig. 13). Ventral curvatures are corrected by removing symmetrical ellipses from the dorsal side of both corpora cavernosa. The dorsal neurovascular bundle has to be carefully mobilized before excising the plaques (Fig. 14); otherwise, damage might be caused to the dorsal arteries, deep dorsal vein, nerves to the glans, and the lymphatics.

In curvatures caused by operative or traumatic scar tissue formation, this dense tissue should be removed or incised before trying to straighten the penis. The ellipsoid openings of the tunica are closed with 3/0 polydioxanone (PDS) (Ethicon) or polyglyconate (Maxon) (Davis and Geck) sutures. These are synthetic, delayed-absorption monofilament sutures. To smoothen the small bumps at the ends of the suture lines, superficial single plicating sutures are made with the same suture material. The artificial erection is then repeated to control the correction, and the penile skin is returned to its normal state and sutured with 3/0 chromic catgut. A silicone foam pressure dressing is placed around the penis: this slightly pressuring dressing prevents the development of edema and he-

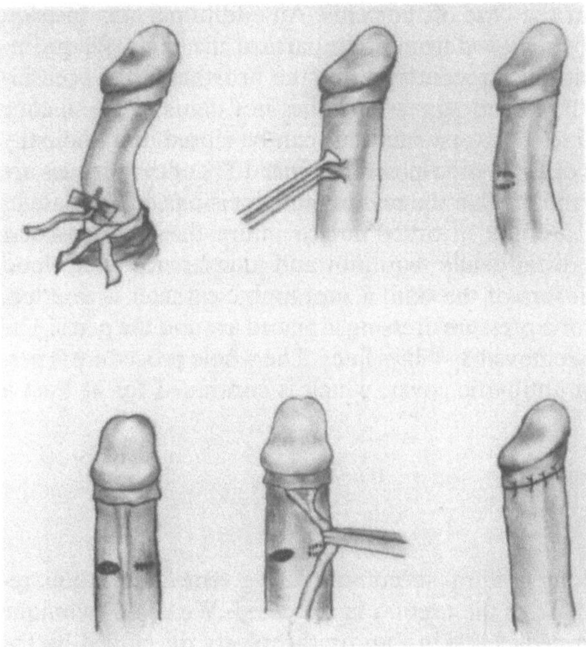

Fig. 14. Nesbit's procedure for ventral curvatures. Note the mobilization of the neurovascular bundle

matoma and is left in place for 3–4 days. Patients are advised to refrain from intercourse for 4–6 weeks.

Penile Prosthesis Implant

For patients with normal erectile function, Nesbit's procedure straightens the penis (Coughlin et al. 1984). For those with impaired erectility accompanying Peyronie's disease or other curvatures, penile prosthesis implant is a rational therapy. The prosthesis splints the deviated penis and also makes penile penetration possible. Insertion of a semirigid rod prosthesis (Raz et al. 1977; Small 1978) or an inflatable prosthesis (Furlow 1978) usually straightens the deviated penis, but when the plaques are hard and the prosthesis cannot straighten the penis, transverse incisions of the plaques help to perfect the penile shape. The problem with the rod prostheses is the permanent erection: even with malleable prostheses of Jonas or AMS-600 type, concealment of the penis becomes a problem some patients complain about. As the inflatable prostheses produce relatively soft erections, they cannot straighten severely deformed penises. Plaque incisions should be made if an inflatable prosthesis is to be inserted, in order to get a good penile shape.

Surgical Technique

The plaque is palpated and the degree of curvature is assessed by creating an artificial erection. We use the infrapubic approach for prosthesis insertion and for plaque incisions that are near the base of the penis. An additional skin incision can be made for plaques to be removed from other parts of the penis. Plaque incisions can be performed with electrocautery after the prosthesis has been inserted. Electrocautery cuts the fibrotic tissue but does not damage the silicone rubber of the prosthesis. These transverse incisions can be closed longitudinally or left open when suturing is difficult or impossible. Since 13% of the plaques are in the intercorporal septum and 55% in the middorsum, incisions of the plaques should be performed very carefully in order not to injure the neurovascular bundle; otherwise, a loss in distal penile sensation and interference with blood supply can develop. After closure of the skin, a suprapubic catheter is inserted, and a silicone foam dressing or a pressure dressing is placed around the penis. The catheter and the dressing are removed 3–4 days later. The whole procedure is performed using wide-spectrum antibiotic cover, which is continued for at least a week.

Urethroplasty

In patients with severe and long urethral strictures causing ventral deviation, reconstruction of the fibrotic part of the urethra is indicated. We use a technique based on the scrotal septum pedicled skin flap urethroplasty developed by the author (Yachia 1986). Patients with severe pendulous urethral strictures who are not inserted in having straight erections can be treated with one of the several urethral patching techniques that repair the stricture but cannot give elasticity to the

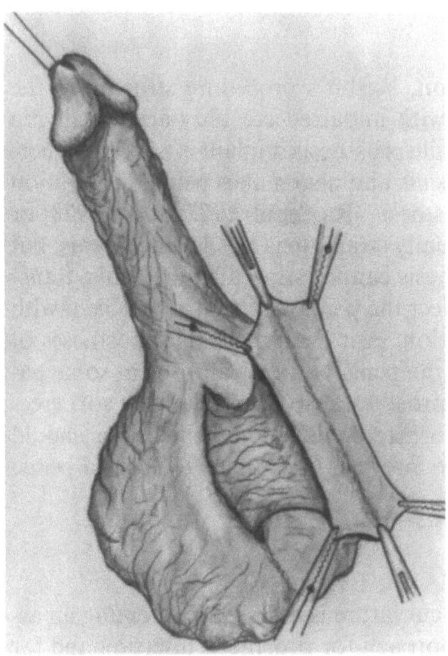

Fig. 15. Preparation of the scrotal septum pedicled skin flap in Yachia's replacement urethroplasty

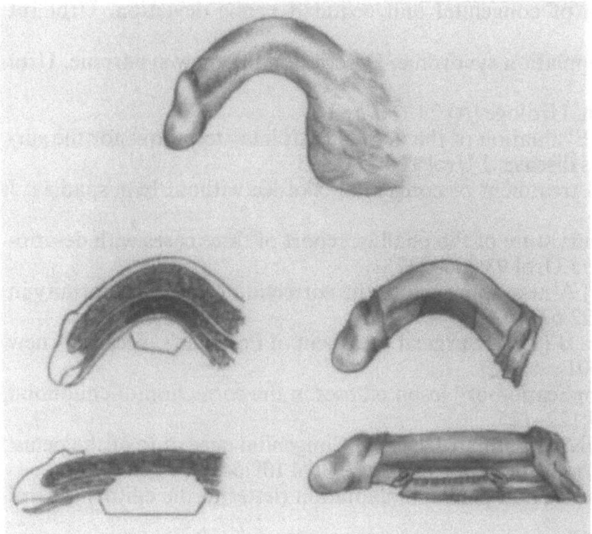

Fig. 16. Yachia's replacement urethroplasty for correction of ventral curvatures caused by urethral manipulations

fibrotic urethra. For those patients who want to be sexually active and have straight erections, reconstruction of a soft urethra is mandatory. For those with impaired erectile function, a penile prosthesis implant is combined with the replacement urethroplasty.

In the urethroplasty technique we developed, a long strip of scrotal skin is prepared along the raphe, leaving it attached to the scrotal septum with its original blood supply (Fig. 15). After resection of the fibrotic part of the urethra, the gap between the healthy ends of the urethra is closed by a tube of the desired length, formed from the prepared flap (Fig. 16). This replacement urethroplasty technique is easy to perform, gives the patient an elastic urethra, and solves the patient's voiding and erectility problems. Unfortunately, the problem of loss of glans engorgement always seen in these patients can no more be solved by this surgical technique than by others.

References

Coughlin PWF, Carson CC, Paulson DF (1984) Surgical correction of Peyronie's disease. Nesbit procedure. J Urol 131:282–284

Das S (1980) Peyronie's disease. Excision and autografting with tunica vaginalis. J Urol 124:818–819

Devine CJ, Horton CE (1974) Surgical treatment of Peyronie's disease. J Urol 111:44–49

Ebbehøj J, Metz P (1985) New operation for "Krummerik" (penile curvature). Urology 26:76–78

Firlow WL (1978) Peyronie's disease and penile implantation (letter to the editor). J Urol 120:647

Hamm B, Friedrich M, Kelâmi A (1986) Ultrasound imaging in Peyronie's disease. Urology 28:540–545

Kelâmi A (1980) Peyronie's disease and surgical treatment. A new concept. Urology 15:559–561

Kelâmi A (1983) Classification of congenital and acquired penile deviation. Urol Int 38:229–233
Kelâmi A (1984) Urethral manipulation syndrome. Description of a new syndrome. Urol Int 39:352–354
Kelâmi A (1985) Penis deviation. Urologe [A] 24:160–163
Melman A, Holland TF (1978) Evaluation of the dermal graft inlay technique for the surgical treatment of Peyronie's disease. J Urol 120:421–423
Nesbit RM (1954) The surgical treatment of congenital chordee without hypospadias. J Urol 72:1178–1180
Nesbit RM (1965) Congenital curvature of the phallus: report of three cases with description of corrective operation. J Urol 93:230–232
Pryor JP, Fitzpatrick JM (1979) A new approach to the correction of penile deformity in Peyronie's disease. J Urol 122:622–623
Raz J, DeKernion JB, Kaufman JJ (1977) Surgical treatment of Peyronie's disease. A new approach. J Urol 117:598–601
Redman JF (1978) Extended application of Nesbit ellipses in the correction of childhood penile curvature. J Urol 119:122–125
Saalfeld J, Ehrlich RM, Grass JM, Kaufman JJ (1973) Congenital curvature of the penis: successful results with variations in corporoplasty. J Urol 109:64–68
Small MP (1978) Peyronie's disease and penile implantation (letter to the editor). J Urol 119:579
Udall DA (1980) Correction of 3 types of congenital curvatures of the penis, including the first reported case of dorsal curvature. J Urol 124:50–52
Yachia D (1986) A new, one-stage pedicled scrotal skin graft urethroplasty. J Urol 136:589–592

Part 3: Neovagina

Surgical Treatment of Vaginal Aplasia: Experience with 134 Cases

Y. Rochet and F. Payan

Gynaecological Department, Université Claude Bernard, Hôpital Edouard Herriot, Place d'Arsonval, 69437 Lyon Cedex 03, France

Our experience of surgical treatment of congenital absence of the vagina comprises 134 cases. We have used most of the technique described hitherto: (a) Frank's nonsurgical method (8 cases); (b) cleavage surgery, either simple or completed by means of a prosthesis or skin grafts (21 cases); (c) transplantation of the intestine (34 cases); and (d) Vecchietti's method (3 cases).

For the past 15 years, we have only used cleavage surgery with two teams (68 cases) because it seems to produce the best results and has the great advantage of being relatively simple and benign. The technique can be used equally well in classic congenital absence of the vagina (Rokitansky's syndrome; 60 cases), congenital absence of the vagina and functional uterus (4 cases), or sexual ambiguities such as male pseudohermaphroditism (4 cases).

Technique

The patient is placed in position for surgery with two teams. A simple , simultaneous cleavage is performed in two directions – from above by the abdominal approach, Pfannenstiel's incision being used in most instances (Fig. 1), and from below by perineal transverse incision (Fig. 2). The greater part of the cleavage is performed by the abdominal team, in the area corresponding to the median peritoneal falcate fold, immediately behind the bladder, which is pushed forward

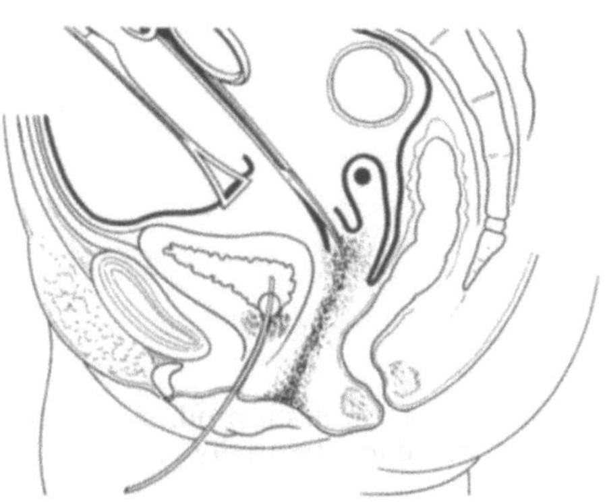

Fig. 1. Pfannenstiel's incision

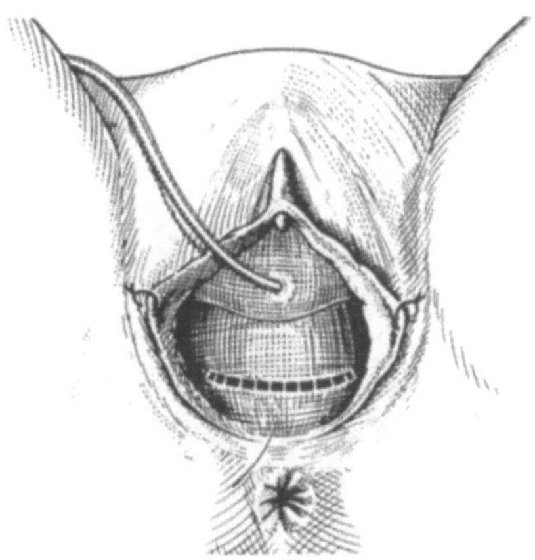

Fig. 2. Perineal transverse incision

Plastic Surgery in the Sexually Handicapped
Eds.: W. Eicher/Kubli/Herms

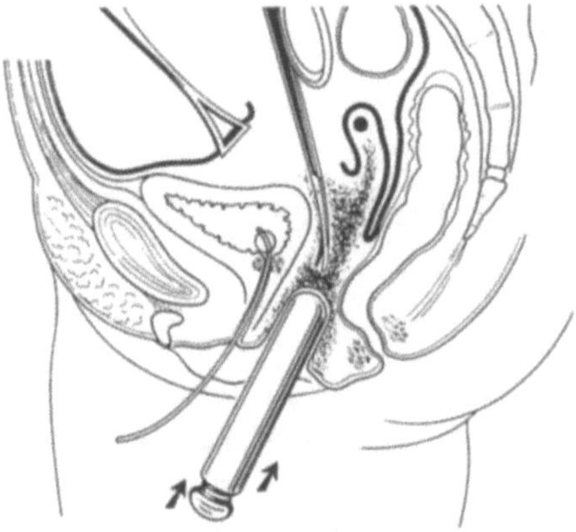

Fig. 3. The bladder is pushed forward as in a hysterectomy

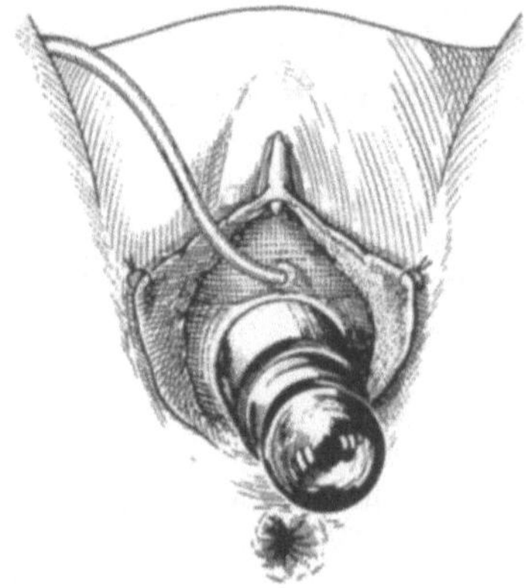

Fig. 4. The tissues are pushed back by means of the dilators introduced from below

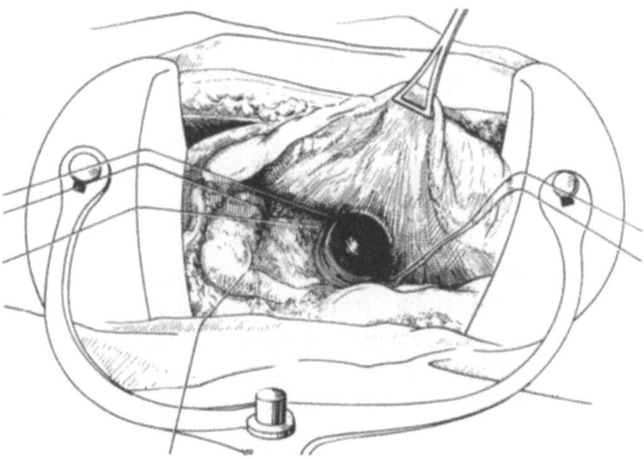

Fig. 5. Cut into the sides

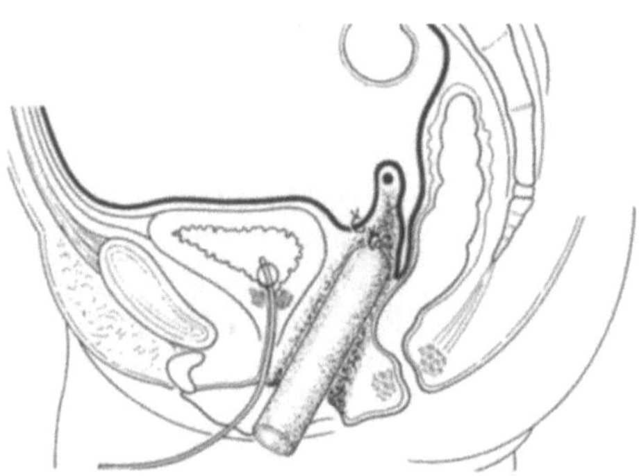

Fig. 6. An elastic prothesis is introduced into the cavity

(Fig. 3) as in a hysterectomy; the cleavage must be extended to a point near the perineal floor.

At this stage, the perineal team penetrates quickly to the space created by the abdominal approach. The few thin tissues are pushed back by means of the established from below (Fig. 4), an incision is made, and communication is established by cutting deeply into the sides (Fig. 5), without going too far because of the passage of the ureters. An elastic, flexible prosthesis 12–15 cm in length by 3–4 cm in thickness is introduced into the cavity thus created (Fig. 6). This prosthesis avoids the risks of possible necrosis of the urethra or rectum, as caused by certain rigid prostheses. The operation ends with the covering of the end of the new vagina, bringing together the vesical peritoneum and the serous top of the median fold.

Postoperative Care

Immediate postoperative care is of the greatest importance and determines long-term success. The sponge prosthesis is left in place for 10–15 days. A second prosthesis is then put in place, and dilations are carried out by means of acrylic mandrels with calibers ranging from 25 to 35 mm. The dilations are performed twice a day, first by the physician and later by the patient herself, who usually understands and accepts the treatment perfectly. A minimum of 4 months must elapse before the results may be considered definite. Epithelialization of the new vagina is monitored by means of cytologic smears. An average of 3 months is necessary for the lower two-thirds of the new vagina to acquire a subnormal cytologic appearance. Intercourse is permitted from the 2nd month.

Indications and Psychological Preparation of Patients

In our opinion and in that of most authors, psychological preparation and precise explanations to the patients are indispensable before surgical treatment is undertaken. We support the idea that the patient must attempt regular sexual activity before being operated on. This is an essential condition for success. Besides, she must know that a pregnancy is not possible.

Results

None of the 68 patients operated on is dead, and there is no significant morbidity. The results are judged according to two criteria, the functional and subjective results by the satisfaction of the patient and partner, and the anatomic result by the length of the vagina as measured by the surgeon.

The latter result is considered to be good if the length is above 7 cm, middling if the vagina measures between 5 and 7 cm, and bad if the length is less than 5 cm and if there is stenosis and/or sclerosis. There is not always a close correlation between the quality of the functional result and that of the anatomic result ; in fact, the surgeon is inclined to severity, while patients are pleased with the results.

Table 1. Results of two-team cleavage operation in 68 patients after 3 months

	Results (no. of patients)		
	Anatomic	Subjective	
Good	56	58	95%
Middling	9	7	
Bad	2	2	4%
No information	1	1	

Table 2. Results of two-team cleavage operation in 68 patients after 1 year

	Results (no. of patients)		
	Anatomic	Subjective	
Good	65	65	98%
Middling	0	0	
Bad	1	1	1%
No information	2	2	

The results are also evaluated as a function of time. After 3 months, we had 65 good or middling results (95% of cases) and 2 failures (4% of cases); we lost track of one patient (Table 1).The psychological behavior of the patients rather than the technique itself is to blame for these failures: these two very young (12-year-old) patients refused to continue dilations. During the 1st year, the most important complications were distal stenosis (8 cases: 11%), always due to lack of daily dilations. The patients were treated with dilations under general anesthesia. Two recurrences were successfully treated by the same technique. After 1 year, the results were better because of the treatment of stenosis, with 65 successful results (98% of cases; Table 2). The results remain excellent many years after the initial operation; we have observed many patients for more than 15 years.

Conclusion

The cleavage operation using two teams making simultaneous abdominal and perineal approaches allows the successful treatment of most malformations with vaginal aplasia. This operation gives pleasure to everybody – patients, partners, and indeed the surgeon; but we must emphasize that if the patient does not want to cooperate, the final result will be a failure, no matter how skillful the surgeon is.

References

Gagnaire JC, Rochet Y (1974) Etude anatomo-clinique des absences congénitals du vagin. J Gynecol Biol Reprod (Paris) 3:415–430

Rochet Y, Dargent D, Vignal J, Conti C, Mathieu J (1970) Grande aplasie cervico-vaginale avec utérus fonctionnel. A propos de deux cas opérés avec succès.) CR Soc Fr Gynécol 6:1–20

Rochet Y, Gagnaire JC et al. (1974) Les aplasies du vagin. Etude des différentes techniques chirurgicales et de leurs résultats. A propos de 57 cas opérés. J Gynecol Obstet Biol Reprod (Paris) 3:223–246

Rochet Y, Bremond A, Rudigoz RC (1983) Les malformations vaginales. In: Encycl Méd Chir, Paris, Techniques Chirurgicales, Urologie-Gynécologie, 4.5.07, 41855

Verbaere S, Rochet Y (1983) Malformations du vagin et de l'hymen. In: Encycl Méd Chir, Paris, Gynécologie, 113 A10, 12-1983

Rochet Y, Gagnaire JC (1975) Treatment of vaginal aplasia by means of cleavage surgery with two teams. Obstet Gynecol Digest 14:13–19

Vecchietti Technique for the Construction of a Neovagina

F. Borruto

Institute of Clinical Obstetrics and Gynecology, University of Verona, Verona, Italy

The Mayer-Rokitansky-Küster (MRK) syndrome, a congenital malformation of the female genitalia (uterus bipartitus solidus rudimentarius cum atresia vaginae), was described by Hauser in 1961 on the basis of analysis of 21 cases from his own experience.

The pathogenesis of the MRK syndrome has not as yet been established. This malformation of the female external genitalia appears to be caused by a teratogenic noxa acting on the embryo during the 2nd month of intrauterine life. Recent discoveries regarding sexual differentiation and the complex enzymatic mechanism, which regulates it, have made it possible to confute the morphogenetic theory held up until only a few years ago. Its exponents regarded the MRK syndrome as an intersexual form and an early stage of female pseudohermaphroditism and true hermaphroditism. Regression of Müller's ducts is certainly a constant element in the abnormal embryogenetic development of this syndrome.

Though modern progress in the early diagnosis of this malformation syndrome has enabled us to diagnose the condition earlier, we believe that the incidence reported by Vecchietti of 1 case in every 5000 births is still a reliable estimate.

Correction of the malformation is surgical. The choice of operation is based on an accurate assessment of the anatomofunctional requirements for the creation of a neovagina with the same characteristics as a normal vagina.

The study population of patients operated on for MRK syndrome by Professor Vecchietti, whom I was fortunate enough to study under, comprises 522 cases over the period from 1962 to 1986. The patients' ages ranged from 14 to 40 years (89 patients aged 14–19, 112 aged 20–24, 243 aged 25–29, 70 aged 30–34, and 8 aged 35–40). None of the patients operated on showed any evidence of major ovarian alterations (cysts, polycysts, etc.). No changes in tubal anatomy were observed, and no complete aplasia of the rudimentary uterus was reported. Urographic evidence of kidney and urinary tract malformation was found in 11 cases (4 cases of aplasia of the right kidney, 2 cases of left kidney ptosis, and 5 cases of pelvic kidney). Account was taken in all cases of the need to operate when the patient expressed a desire to have a normal sex life.

Vecchietti's operative technique utilizes the following instruments: a straight suture needle, a curved suture needle, an acrylic olive with attached nonabsorbable suture threads (Mersilene; Perlon, silk), a spring-operated traction device, and phantom phalluses of various lengths and calibers.

The patient is placed on the operating table with her legs slightly apart, and with a narrow-caliber Foley bladder catheter inserted. A Pfannenstiel incision is

Plastic Surgery in the Sexually Handicapped
Eds.: W. Eicher/Kubli/Herms

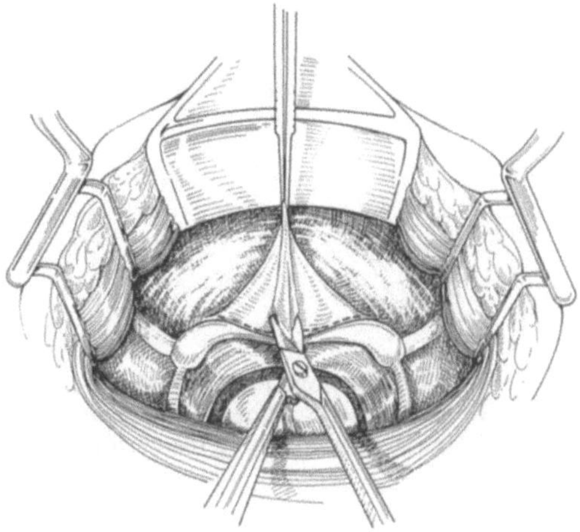

Fig. 1. The vesicouterine peritoneal fold is raised and a transverse incision is made

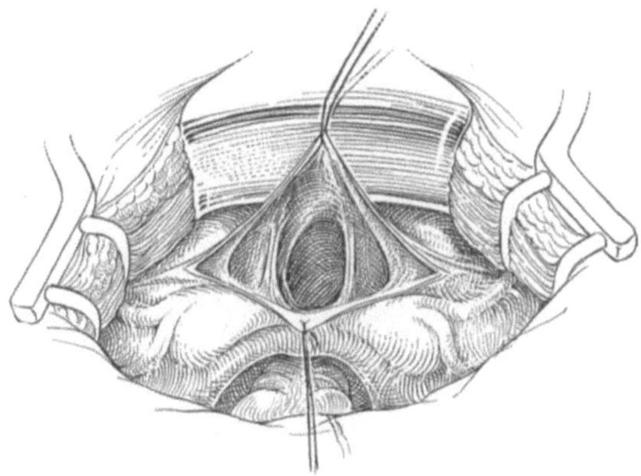

Fig. 2. Intervesicourethrorectal tunnel

made, taking care to extend it laterally beyond the rectus muscles. With the abdominal cavity open, a suture thread or clamp is attached to the midpoint of the intrauterine ligament, the vesicouterine peritoneal fold is raised, and a transverse incision of approximately 4–5 cm is made (Fig. 1). Bevel-edged forceps are used to create an intervesicourethrorectal tunnel via a cleavage plane easily traceable as far as the pseudohymenal membrane (Fig. 2). The upper part of this tunnel presents small connective formations consisting of rudimentary uterovesical ligaments. If the cleavage plane is the right one, the walls of the neovaginal canal will be exsanguine.

The straight suture needle is introduced into the tunnel, being controlled from the outside by the operator's finger, which presses the center of the pseudohymenal membrane inwards, guiding the perforation (Fig. 3). The integrity of the rectum must be checked by rectal exploration. (Rectal lesions occurred in only one case in our study population.) This maneuver is facilitated by the presence of the suture needle. The threads of the olive are passed through the eye of the suture needle, which is then pulled back, drawing the threads through the newly formed tunnel into the abdominal cavity (Figs. 4, 5). Bladder integrity is checked by introducing a solution of methylene blue via the catheter. A curved suture nee-

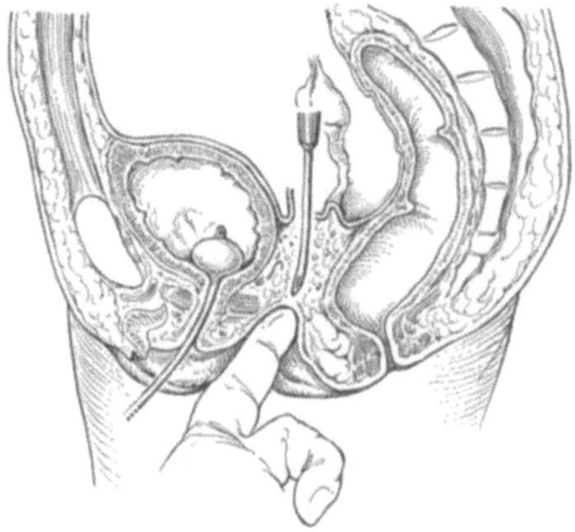

Fig. 3. Operator's finger presses the center of the pseudohymenal membrane inwards, guiding the perforation

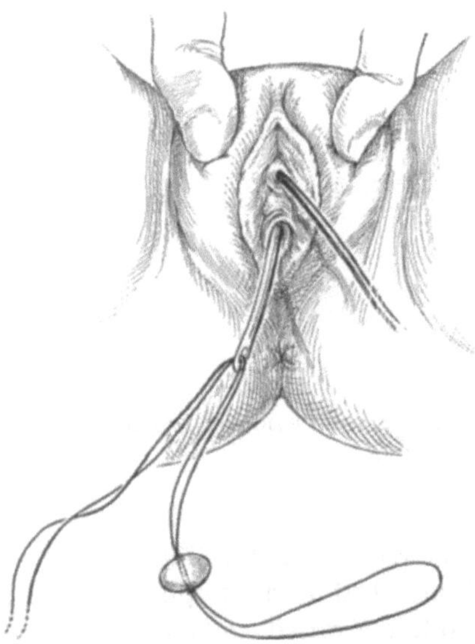

Fig. 4. The threads and the olive are drawn into the abdominal cavity

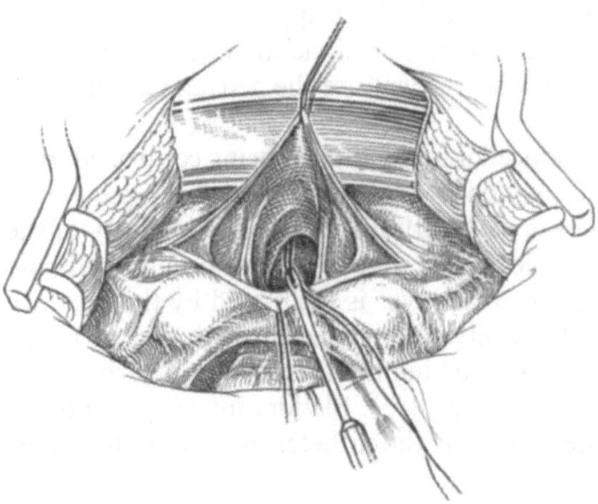

Fig. 5. The threads are drawn into the abdominal cavity through the newly formed tunnel

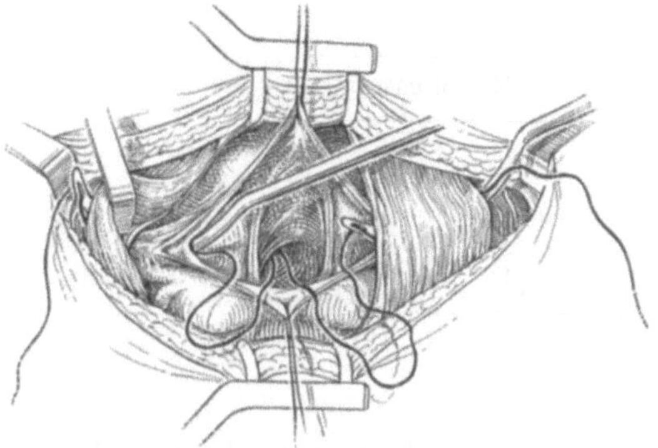

Fig. 6. The curved surture needle is following the round ligaments and brings the threads subperitoneally through the abdominal walls

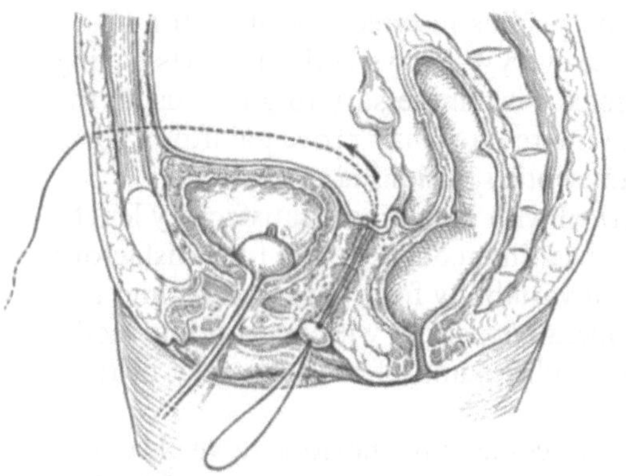

dle is inserted at the end of the Pfannenstiel incision and – taking care to penetrate midway between the lower epigastric vessels – is slipped laterally below first the lateral and then the visceral peritoneal wall, following a path caudal to the round ligaments, as far as the lateral corner on each side of the incision in the vesicouterine fold (Fig. 6). This maneuver is facilitated by medial stretching of the round ligaments. The threads are picked up, drawn along subperitoneally, and then brought to the surface bilaterally. The incisions in the perivesical peritoneum and in the abdominal walls are sutured.

The threads are attached to an adjustable spring-operated traction device. The traction force must be appropriately gauged to avoid lacerating the dome of the vagina. This can be checked by finger pressure on the bottom end of the olive, which should allow an elastic upward displacement of about 1 cm. The traction force on the threads will be adjusted daily so as to produce a progressive upward displacement of the olive and thus a lengthening of the vagina (Fig. 7). As a rule, the length of the vagina increases to 11–12 cm in 7–8 days. More rapid results are achieved in younger women owing to the greater elasticity of the tissues.

The olive is removed by cutting the threads at skin level and pulling the trailing threads out via the vulva. The catheter is removed, and a phantom phallus is introduced. The latter measures 11–12 cm in length and 2–2.5 cm in diameter, is smeared with antibiotic cream, and is held in place by elastic pants. Tolerance

Table 1. Complications

Complication	No. of cases
Perforation of bladder	1
Perforation of rectum	1
Hemorrhage of dome of vagina	3
Cystitis	3
Rectovaginal fistula	1

of the phallus is checked for a few days, after which the patient is discharged from hospital.

At home, the patient should keep the phallus inserted overnight for 10–15 days; thereafter, it should be inserted once every 4–5 days until she starts having sexual intercourse, which, if frequent, makes it unnecessary to go on using the phallus. The first few attempts at sexual intercourse may prove painful in some patients. Daily vaginal irrigation with antiseptic solutions is advisable.

The operator should be more concerned with obtaining a satisfactory length than with the diameter of the vagina. Sexual intercourse makes for satisfactory results. There is, of course, a great deal of variability from case to case, and this must be borne in mind during the postoperative period, with appropriate modifications of the length and diameter of phalluses and of the frequency of their use.

All patients operated on were invited to come in for postoperative checkups after 1 month, 3 months, 1 year, and 2 years. All patients came in for the first checkup after 1 month, while only 30% reported for the 2-year checkup.

At the checkup after 1 month, a certain number of patients, i.e., between 12% and 15%, reported the occurrence of dyspareunia; this had disappeared by the time of the 3-month checkup. In two patients aged 14 and 15 years respectively, continuous phallotherapy was needed owing to the absence of sexual intercourse. These two patients, operated on in 1979 and 1980 respectively, came in for a checkup several years later (end of 1985), and we found that the neovagina had reached a substantial length owing to the breaching of the dome of the vagina as a result of pressure exerted by the phallus.

In eight of the patients treated, the dome-breaching complication was the result of excessive traction on the olive postoperatively.

In one case, a patient operated on in 1983, the complication observed was a rectovaginal fistula. We believe this complication was due to improper use of the phantom phallus. The fistula was successfully treated without difficulty when the patient elected to undergo a second operation some 3 years later.

The anatomical characteristics of the neovagina are the same as those of normal vaginal mucosa. In only one case did the patient (aged 32 years when operated on) refuse to accept the neovagina owing to preexisting psychological problems. This patient chose, of her own free will, to have no sexual intercourse. The neovagina, though narrow, showed no sign of loss of tone or tendency to close up.

In two cases, there were perioperative lesions of the rectum and bladder, respectively, in the form of perforations caused by the straight suture needle. These perforations were promptly diagnosed, and the suture needle was reinserted in the correct cleavage plane; no aftereffects or complications were observed. Two patients in our study population presented a Morris syndrome, the creation of the neovagina being accompanied by gonadectomy.

References

Borruto F (1982) Sexualität nach operierter Vaginalaplasie. Sexualmedizin 11:476–477
Golditch IM (1969) Vaginal aplasia. Surg Gynecol Obstet 123:461–466
Hauser GA, Schreiner WE (1961) Das Mayer-Rokitansky-Küster Syndrom. Schweiz Med Wochenschr 12:381–391
Käser O (1987) Atlante di chirurgia ginecologica. Cortina, Verona pp 1417–1420
Richter K, Terruhn V (1982) Zur klinischen Anatomie der Aplasia vaginae. Morphol Med 2:81–97
Rochet Y (1982) La technique de Vecchietti. In: Encyclopédie Medico-Chirurgicale Mason, Paris
Rochet Y, Gagneire JC (1974) Les aplasies du vagin – Etude des différentes techniques chirurgicales et de leurs résultats. J Gynecol Obstet Biol Reprod 3:223–246
Vecchietti G (1965) Neovagina nella sindrome di Rokitansky-Küster-Hauser. Attual Ost Ginecol 11:131
Vecchietti G (1979) Le néovagin dans la syndrome de Rokitansky-Küster-Hauser. Rev Med Suisse Romande 99:593
Vecchietti G, Ardillo L (1970) La sindrome di Rokitansky-Küster-Hauser. SEU, Rome
Vecchietti G (1980) Die Neovagina beim Rokitansky-Küster-Hauser Syndrom. Gynäkologie 13:112–115
Vecchietti G, Borruto F (1985) The retaining and restoring of sexual function by means of gynecologic surgery. In: Segraves Taylor R, Haeberle E (eds) Emerging dimensions of sexology. Praeger, New York

Peritoneal Colpopoiesis

S. N. Davydov

Postgraduate Medical Institute, Saltynova-Str. 41, Leningrad, USSR, 1930JS
Department of Obstetrics and Gynecology,
Leningrad Institute for Advanced Medical Training of Physicians. Leningrad, 193015 USSR

All the presently existing methods of vagina formation may be divided into three groups: (a) colpopoiesis without the application of surgical methods ("bloodless method"); (b) colpopoiesis utilizing stretches of different sections of the intestine; and (c) colpopoiesis with the application of plastic interventions, including auto- and homoplasty, and alloplasty (heteroplasty).

It should be said that autoplastic methods play the leading role in dealing with the problem of colpopoiesis. Evidently, as will be seen further on, it is necessary to continue the search for those materials which – on the basis of their properties and anatomical peculiarities, the safety of their utilization, and the final results – would give the very best results.

The first reference to the possibility of transferring the peritoneum of the small pelvis into an artificially formed canal between the urinary bladder and rectum is made in the works of the well-known Russian gynecologist D. O. Ott, who performed such an operation in 1897; however, he did not report on the results.

In 1933, a Russian gynecologist, M. G. Ksido, reported on an operation in which the peritoneum of the small pelvis was used for colpopoiesis. The result of the operation was quite satisfactory. From this time on, reports of peritoneal colpopoiesis began to appear in print. At present we have data on vagina formation from the peritoneum performed in more than 1200 women in various clinics in the USSR, Europe, and the United States. Moreover, all the authors report entirely satisfactory results.

Up until 1970, the method of peritoneal colpopoiesis consisted of two stages. The first of these included the formation of a canal between the urethra, urinary bladder, and rectum, and the insertion of a tampon. The second stage included laparatomy, during which the peritoneum was incised above the tampon, and its edges were brought down to the entrance into the vagina; then, the bottom of the abdominal cavity was formed. Since 1970, we have introduced a significant modification: a one-stage peritoneal approach has been studied.

Two-Stage Colpopoiesis Technique

In the two-stage method, the mucous membrane of the vaginal entrance was distended with forceps and dissected in a lateral direction (Fig. 1). The tissue between the urinary bladder and the rectum was dissected, partly by the sharp and partly by the blunt method, and the canal thus formed was firmly packed with tampons (Fig. 2). The tampon packing played a double role: it controlled tissue bleeding

Plastic Surgery in the Sexually Handicapped
Eds.: W. Eicher/Kubli/Herms

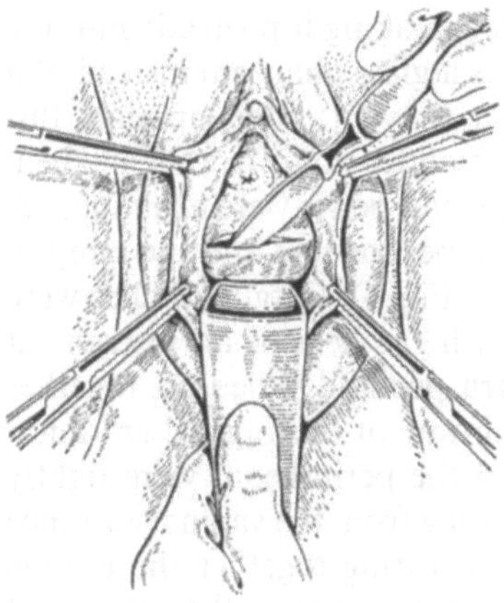

Fig. 1. Transverse incision and dissection Between bladder and rectum

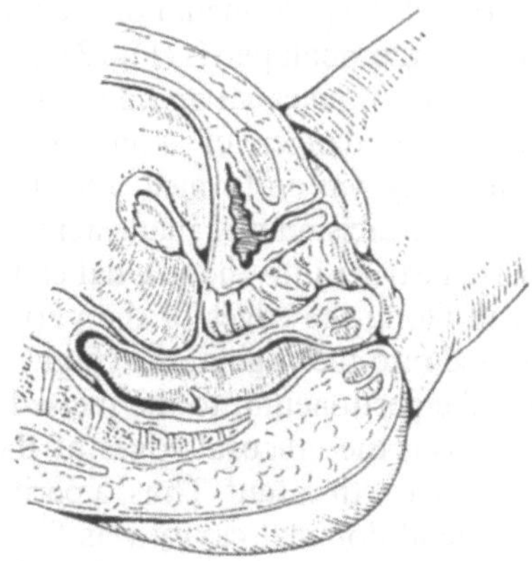

Fig. 2. Canal between bladder and rectum packed with tampons

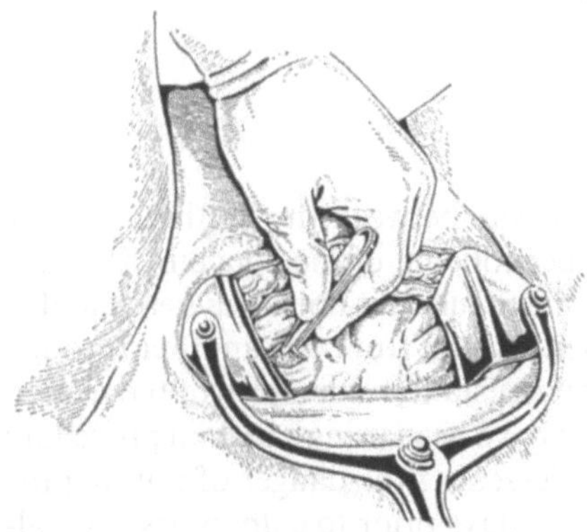

Fig. 3. Transverse incision across the protruding peritoneum above the tampon

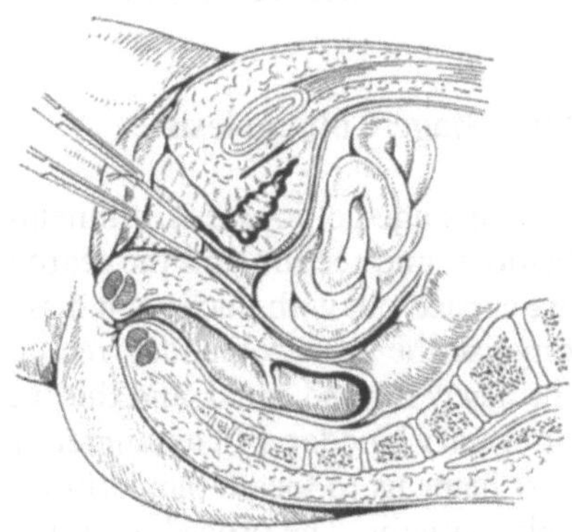

Fig. 4. Peritoneum is pulled down and tightly connected with catgut to the edges of the vaginal entrance

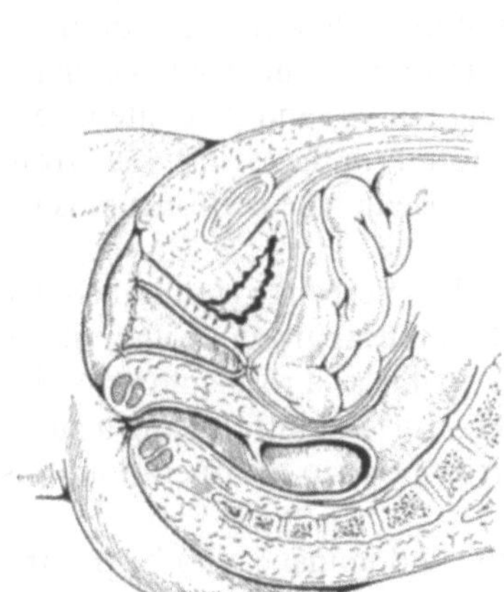

Fig. 5. Closing new vaginal vault by suture

and raised the peritoneum of the pouch of Douglas, making it protrude into the cavity of the small pelvis (Fig. 3). (Friedberg inserts a glass phantom instead of a tampon into the canal and dissects the peritoneum above it: in his opinion, this lessens the danger of wounding the urinary bladder and rectum.) Then, laparotomy was performed, and the organs of the small pelvis were examined. A transverse incision was made across the protruding peritoneum and the tampon inserted earlier into the vaginal canal was revealed (Fig. 4). Catgut stitches were put in along the edges of the peritoneum, and with the help of an instrument inserted into the vagina; the catgut sutures were grasped and pulled up, together with the peritoneum, to the incised mucous membrane of the vaginal entrance. Here also, the mucosal edges of the entrance and the peritoneum were tightly connected with catgut. Thus, a peritoneal tube running from the vaginal entrance into the abdominal cavity was formed. Then, by suturing together the uterine rudiments and sacrouterine folds of the peritoneum, the bottom of the abdominal cavity was formed; in addition, the anterior wall of the rectum was attached to this last suture. In this way, the abdominal cavity was separated from the newly formed vagina (Fig. 5). When the laparotomy was concluded, an oily, antiseptic tampon was inserted into the artificial vagina.

One-Stage Colpopoiesis

In one-stage colpopoiesis, tunneling of the tissue between the urethra, urinary bladder, and rectum and the search for the peritoneum of the pouch of Douglas are carried out with maximum dissection of the tissue. It is not always easy to distinguish the urinary bladder, rectum, and peritoneum from one another through the newly formed canal, and this may lead to a mistake, with injury of the rectum or urinary bladder. For a number of years, we have been using a certain procedure that helps us to locate the peritoneum, thus lessening the danger of injuring the pelvic organs. The procedure is as follows: 2–3 days prior to colpopoiesis, we always perform a pelviographic examination in order to establish the diagnosis of uterine aplasia. This examination, of courses requires the administration of gas into the abdominal cavity. The development of pneumoperitoneum always leads to the appearance of an increased quantity of peritoneal fluid in the abdominal cavity, which we deal with in the following way: as soon as the vaginal canal is formed, the presumed site of the peritoneum is punctured, and its contents are drawn off. If a yellowish liquid appears in large amounts in the syringe (i.e., from the abdominal cavity), then, without extracting the needle, the peritoneum is incised, and its edges are grasped with instruments.

In order to facilitate this stage of the operation, Dr. Verbenko simultaneously explores the peritoneum by laparoscopy. The bulb of the laparoscope illuminates the thin peritoneum quite well; the latter becomes visible as a rose-colored "window" at the depth of the canal. Another method consists of introducing a small amount of methylene blue into the abdominal cavity prior to the operation; this dyes the peritoneum, making it easier to locate.

The newly formed vagina is separated from the abdominal cavity by putting in one catgut pursestring suture in the depth of the vaginal tube. The operation is concluded by inserting an oily, antiseptic tampon. Immediately after the operation, some surgeons (e.g., Willemsen) insert a rigid mold into the newly formed vagina and keep it there for several days; we do not find this necessary. The tampon in the vagina is first changed on the 3rd postoperative day. Later on, the tampons are changed every other day.

In order to promote healing, it is beneficial to include estrogens in the oil mixtures.

At the first change of tampon, the peritoneum was bright red and edematous with slight fibrinogenous deposits (coating); i.e., it presented an inflamed appearance, as in peritonitis. As the postoperative period increased, the edema decreased, and the peritoneum acquired a pink, and then a whitish color and became paler than the mucosa of the vaginal entrance.

The borderline between the peritoneum and the mucosa of the entrance was always distinctly seen. A close, compact connection of the edges of the two tissues set in by the 7th–8th day; by this time, the connecting catgut sutures had dissolved. The entrance mucosa always turned out to extend beyond the site where it was initially located, and thus it became part of the general vaginal tube.

Cytological studies of vaginal discharge and histological studies of pieces of the vaginal tube carried out during the first days of the postoperative period confirmed the presence of an inflammatory process in the transferred peritoneum.

The patients were discharged on the 15th–16th postoperative day. Sexual intercourse was permitted 5–8 days after discharge. If the patient did not have the possibility to have sexual intercourse, she was recommended to use a prosthesis during the first 1.5–2 months, which was to be kept inserted in the artificial vagina overnight. Postoperative Complications are shown in Table 1.

The results were followed up in 188 women during the period from 1 to 15 years postoperatively: 150 women led a regular sexual life, 32 had irregular coitus, and 6 patients had sexual intercourse very rarely. Only 2 patients complained that they found sexual intercourse painful, 128 women experienced orgasm, and the only complaint on the part of the husbands was absence of pregnancy. The fact that only 32 sexual partners knew that the woman had undergone some vaginal surgical intervention presents a certain interest.

Data from written reports and direct studies revealed that neither the method nor time has any significant influence upon the dimensions of the vagina. The

Table 1. Postoperative complications (432 operations)

Complication	No. of cases	
	Two-stage method	One-stage method
Suppuration of the operative wound	4	0
Thrombophlebitis of the lower extremities	1	2
Paresis of the intestine	7	4
Pelvioperitonitis	0	2
Prolonged fever	6	8
Cystitis	9	9
Lethal outcome	0	0

one-stage method is better tolerated by the patients, but it is necessary to know how to perform the two-stage method as well since it must be used in cases of tumor in the small pelvis, in obese women, and also in learning the technique of peritoneal colpopoiesis.

In examining the vagina during long-term follow-up, it was nearly always possible to locate the border between the entrance and the former peritoneum by the paler color of the latter. The vagina was satisfactorily moistened. Vaginography carried out in all patients during examination in the clinic revealed that the vagina was equally wide along its whole length.

During our observation of the women, we carried out bacteriological studies, which in some patients revealed growth of *Staphylococcus albus*, rarer streptococci and *Escherichia coli*. Colpocytological studies carried out immediately after the operation revealed a clearly defined inflammatory reaction, with destruction of peritoneal mesothelium; after 2 months, only cells of stratified squamous epithelium were found. In a number of cases, it was possible to correlate the changes in the cytological reaction to the phases of the menstrual cycle.

Histological studies of the vaginal walls carried out at the end of the 1st postoperative week disclosed necrosis and acute inflammation, tissue destruction, and leukocyte infiltration; there was also fibroblast proliferation and new formation of vessels. Then a picture characteristic of granular tissue formation emerged. Three weeks later, epithelization of the artificial vagina surface was observed, but it was accompanied by growth of stratified squamous epithelium of the vaginal entrance mucosa.

In summary, the inflammatory-destructive processes are followed by a restoration of anatomical conditions similar to those in a normal vagina, excluding the muscular elements in the latter.

The performance of urography before an operation is essential, and if a single kidney shift into the small pelvis is detected peritoneal colpopoiesis will be contraindicated since apicolysis of the peritoneum may bring about a dangerous displacement of the kidney.

Evaluation of the various methods of colpopoiesis is, in the long run, based upon the functional completeness of the neovagina. Consideration of the result of a peritoneal colpopoiesis shows that the neovagina turns out to be of full value, providing a normal sexual life and normal sexual sensations for the couple.

References

Davydov SN (1977) Abdominal Colpopoiesis. Leningrad Medizina

Davydov SN, Chromow BM, Scheiko WZ (1982) Atlas of gynecological operations. 2nd edition. Leningrad Medizina

Part 4: Vaginal Repair

Surgical Treatment of Sexual Dysfunction – The Lost Penis Syndrome

C. Debrovner 165 West End Ave, New York, NY 10023, USA

Though surgery does have a place in the management of sexual dysfunction, the message of this contribution is that it should be the treatment of last resort, utilized only when all other modalities of therapy have proved to be unsuccessful.

Disproportion between the size of the vagina and the size of the penis can cause coital difficulties for both men and women. In young women, the vagina generally contracts to fit the penis. Masters and Johnson have emphasized this point in their effort to teach that the size of the penis is a relatively unimportant factor. The healthy vagina makes compensations to bring about good contact between the two mucous membranes for adequate friction. If adequate vaginal compensation does not occur, both partners suffer: for the man, there may be virtually no gripping or sensation of penetration, with a resultant decrease in friction from intercourse; for the woman, because the penis is not tightly gripped, there is decreased movement of the labia minora, which at their upper margin form the frenulum and prepuce of the clitoris and transmit stimulation to it. This results in decreased clitoral stimulation and orgasmic dysfunction; in addition, there is a general loss of a feeling of vaginal distention and the pleasant stimulation of friction.

In evaluating this complaint, care must be taken to be sure that it is of anatomic origin. Therapy designed to correct an anatomic defect will not improve a sexual relationship problem. On the other hand, marriage counselling will not improve a nonfunctioning or severely damaged pubococcygeal muscle. A detailed sexual history and careful vaginal examination are necessary to select the approach or combination of approaches that best meets the couple's need.

Much of the physical pleasure and sensation of intercourse is derived from friction. Factors resulting in a decrease in friction that are other than truly anatomic may be both exogenous and endogenous. Excessive use of lubricants or the lubricating effect of contraceptive creams and jellies may decrease sensation. Excessive vaginal discharge, perhaps related to a chronic cervicitis, may similarly decrease friction. Modifications in this area should not prove to be too difficult.

Another factor to be considered is that many older men sustain much less firm erections than they did in their youth. This means that the penis is smaller at the same time that the vagina may be larger. One way in which the mature woman can help compensate for this discrepancy is to be more active in stimulating her husband, rather than assuming the more passive role that she might have played in her youth. Similarly, the husband may have to spend more time in foreplay since his wife may take longer to be aroused. Arousal is important in producing vaginal contractions, thereby compensating for some of the stretching. Thus, it

Plastic Surgery in the Sexually Handicapped
Eds.: W. Eicher/Kubli/Herms

is important for an older couple to take equal responsibility for finding method of keeping each other sexually responsive and satisfied.

Several physical means can be used to increase friction. Direct digital clitoral stimulation by either partner with the couple lying on their side during intercourse can frequently provide increased pleasure for the woman. Either partner can direct the erect penis against a particular area of the vagina; angling the penis in such a way that the glans is directed against the anterior vaginal wall is frequently helpful. Insertion from behind can accomplish this as well. The woman can taken one or both of her hands and stretch the skin at the base of the penis against the man's pubis, thereby increasing the sensation on the stretched glans, or she can place her hands on the shaft of the penis near its base and, by varying pressure, simulate vaginal barrel friction. Similarly, pressure along the lateral aspects of the labia against the shaft of the penis can enhance sensation for both partners.

Male impotence may really be involved in a small subgroup of patients presenting initially with this complaint. As a gynecologist, I will not discuss this group at great length, but merely say that in the great majority of these men, the problem was psychogenic. However, I may mention that in cases of organic impotence as well as those cases where the psychogenic problem is so severe that therapy is unsuccessful, there has been successful use of penile prostheses to correct the problem.

Gynecological evaluation of the female partner will often show a parous woman whose labia gape, barely covering the vaginal introitus, and whose anterior and/or posterior vaginal walls bulge through the opening, forming a cystocele or rectocele, with a lack of turgor, color, and normal rugal formation. There may be perineal defects from poorly healed episiotomy scars, especially those of the medial-lateral variety. Such findings strongly suggest that the problem has a female anatomic origin and demand an anatomic solution. This solution may take the form of restoration of altered muscle physiology or surgical correction. In either case, the key to the solution is that muscle which is most intimately related to the status of the vaginal introitus and the distal one-third of the vagina, that portion of the levator ani muscle known as the pubococcygeus.

Fibers of this muscle can be torn or severely stretched during childbirth. In many women, when estrogen levels are high and the tone and strength of the remaining muscle fibers is good, the loss of part of the muscle can be compensated for. As time goes on – with progressive aging, further childbirth, and loss of estrogen – this compensation is no longer possible, and the structures supported by this muscle begin to sag, with resultant loss of introital and vaginal tone, and often, secondary descensus of uterus, bladder, and rectum. In some women, the ability to contract these muscles voluntarily has never been successfully acquired, and even in the absence of childbirth, the muscles lack tone and are poorly developed.

As early as 1952, Kegel reported that observations concerning the sexual properties of the pubococcygeus indicated the presence of two distinct but interrelated functions: (a) distinct sphincteric actions and (b) sensory perception. The latter is probably accomplished through specialized proprioceptors closely related to awareness of muscle function. He went on to say that the sphincteric and sensory sexual function of the vagina is practically always potentially present and can be developed through muscle education and resistive exercise. Every woman with sexual complaints should be investigated for possible dysfunction of the pubococcygeus. In a large percentage of cases, it will be found that lack of vaginal feeling and so-called frigidity can be traced to faulty development of function of this muscle.

Kegel reported that his studies, begun in 1932, had been incidental to efforts to improve the ultimate results of vaginal plastic surgery. In the course of those efforts, he had developed a perineometer since he found that women who possess awareness of function of the vaginal muscles are able to carry out active exercises once they have been carefully instructed. Those who lack initial awareness of function require muscle education and progressive resistive exercise with the aid of this device.

In my own experience, the diagnosis of levator muscle dysfunction can be made by an exercise performed in the examining room: the patient is instructed to pretend that she is urinating, that the telephone rings, and that she must stop urinating in order to answer the telephone. She is instructed to contract those muscles which are necessary for her to stop urinating. Generally, this sets up sufficiently familiar pathways for the patient to be able to contract this muscle, and its tone can be evaluated by palpating it vaginally. If the woman is unable to contract this muscle or contracts it poorly, she is instructed to establish the pathway initially by stopping the urinary stream at home. Once she has developed the ability to do so, she can then continue to contract the muscle frequently throughout the day – independently of urination – either in short, frequent contractions or in long-sustained contractions. She then returns periodically for evaluation of her progress.

Frequently, the use of systemic or topical estrogen will greatly improve the function of this muscle, and in suitable candidates, I have not found the use of a mechanical device such as a perineometer to be necessary. It is only when all of the above modifications in sexual technique and efforts to restore muscle function physiologically have failed that one should resort to surgery.

The surgical procedure performed is not appreciably different from that which is utilized in standard vaginal plastic operations. However, there are two major goals when the procedure is performed specifically for sexual dysfunction: (a) to restore the integrity of the perineum and hence decrease the size of the vaginal introitus, and, most importantly, (b) to bring together the fibers of the pubococcygeus in the midline between the vagina and rectum, thereby shortening them, tightening them, and improving their ability to function. This surgical procedure may then be coupled with the use of perineal exercises afterward. One should take care not to be overzealous in attempts to correct this problem. Such attempts may so tighten the entrance to the vagina that the older male partner, with an erection of diminished firmness, is unable to penetrate it.

In conclusion, the need to perform surgical correction of pubococcygeal muscle dysfunction is inversely proportional to the enthusiasm of the therapist for Kegel's exercises and other modalities for correction of sexual dysfunction by reorientation of sexual partners; however, when the surgical procedure is performed in appropriately selected patients, the results are quite good. I wish to stress the importance of the selection of patients and reiterate that surgery will no more improve a sexual relationship problem than marriage counselling will improve non-functioning or severely damaged pelvic anatomy.

References

Kegel AH (1952) Sexual functions of the pubococcygeus muscle. West J Obstet Gynecol October 1952, p 521

Masters Wh, Johnson VE (1966) Human sexual response. Little Brown Comp Publ Boston Mass

Masters Wh, Johnson VE (1970) Human sexual inadequacy. Little Brown Comp Publ Boston Mass

Part 5: Genital Transformation

Vaginoplasty, with Abdominally Pedicled Penis Skin in Male-to-Female, Transsexuals

F. G. Bouman

Department of Plastic and Reconstructive Surgery,
Academisch Ziekenhuis Vrije Universiteit, de Boelelaan 1117, 1081 HV Amsterdam,
Netherlands

Several techniques have been described for transforming, the external genitalia of a male transsexual in the female direction. Nearly all these techniques make use of the penis skin or scrotal skin flaps to cover the dissected vaginal cavity with epithelium. With a pedicle flap that has its own circulation, there is no risk of a stricture; however, a process of scarring can be initiated by a hematoma, or if too much damage has been done to the surrounding tissues in preparing the cavity. Fistula from the rectum or bladder will not occur either, if there is a good circulation in the skin flaps. In transsexuals, other methods, such as the use of split skin, rectosigmoid, or peritoneum, are only used in cases of total failure of the primary operation. There are three main principles: (a) use of the inverted penile skin tube on an abdominal pedicle (Stuteville et al. 1971), (b) the same, but on a caudal pedicle (Edgerton and Bull 1970), and (c) use of the penile skin as a flap, together with a caudally, pedicled scrotal flap (Jones et al. 1968).

I used the first principle, described in 1971 by Stuteville et al. Since 1980 more than 70 male-to-female transsexuals have been operated on in this way. (A follow-up study of 55 of these patients will be published in *Annals of Plastic Surgery*.)

In my opinion, the advantages of this technique are (a) the circulation in the penile skin flap is good, (b) the appearance of the result is good, (c) the vagina is hairless, and (d) the results can be obtained in one operation. The main drawbacks of this technique are (a) the depth and width of the vagina are dependent on the available penis skin tube, though in my experience a depth of 10 cm can always be reached, and (b) traction has to be placed on the abdominal pedicle to move the penile skin towards the vaginal opening. This traction does not impair the circulation in my experience, but it can give a skin fold on the posterior wall of the introitus vaginae.

Technique

The patient is placed in the lithotomy position. The incision is made in the shape of an inverted Y. It starts as a median incision at the base of the penis, more than 10 cm from the corona, passes through the raphe scroti, and divides at the base of the scrotum into two diverging lines ending in the perineum (Fig. 1). In this way, a caudally based perineal flap is formed, which can be used to widen the introitus. The tubular dissection of the penis skin is facilitated by injection of local anesthetic [0.5% lidocaine (Xylocaine) and 1:200000 epinephrine (Adrenalin)]. A coronal incision is made, and the contents of the penis are pulled out of the skin

Plastic Surgery in the Sexually Handicapped
Eds.: W. Eicher/Kubli/Herms

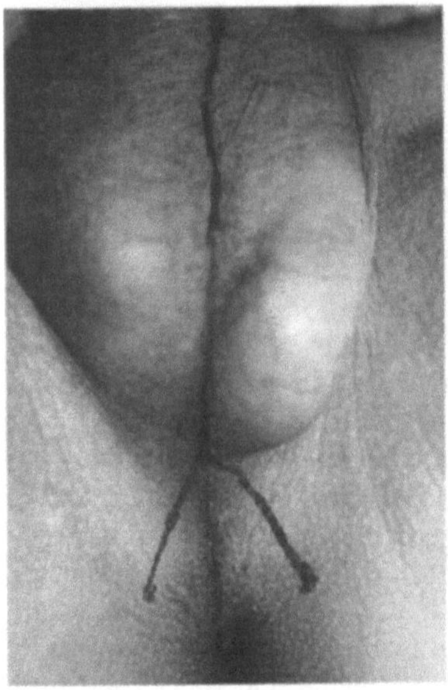

Fig. 1. Incision lines for the formation of a caudally based perineal flap

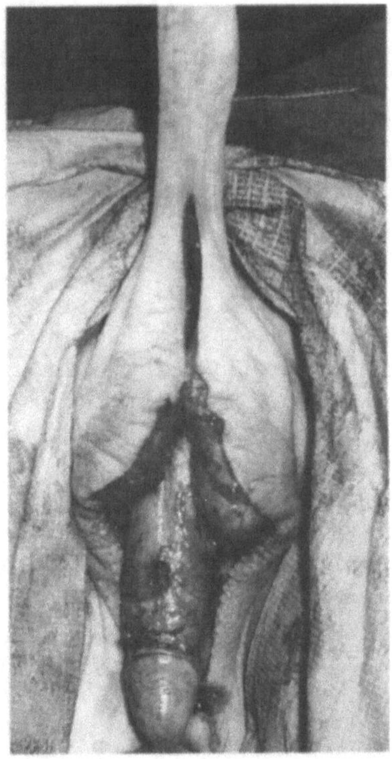

Fig. 2. Penis separated from its skin envelope

envelope (Fig. 2). The top of the penis skin will be closed. The testicles are freed from the surrounding tissue with a diathermic knife. The funiculi spermatici are clamped and cut just above the testicles and closed with a transfixing ligature.

On the dorsal side, the dorsal vessels and nerves are cut through 5 cm from the base and dissected from the corpora cavernosa in a flap to the base. The top of this flap will be laid on the symphysis at the point where the clitoris should be situated.

The urethra with its corpus spongiosum is isolated from the corpora 5 cm above the trigonum urogenitale and is cut (Fig. 3). After inserting a metal probe in ther urethra, the urethra is separated from both corpora down to the trigonum (septum urogenitale). The crura are isolated as far as their origin at the ramus inferior ossis pubis. They are clamped, cut, and closed with a transfixing ligature. If more room is needed, complete removal of the origins is also possible. The contents of the penis can now be taken out.

The next step is removal of the corpus spongiosum from the urethra, which is not so easy: the urethra is very thin and fragile, and bleeding from the erectile body makes removal difficult. Behind the urethra and the trigonum, a cavity has to be made in the septum rectovesicale (Denonvilliers' fascia), using the metal probe in the urethra as a guide. In the midline, a fibrous connection between the trigonum and the sphincter ani has to be cut. When one has found the right space,

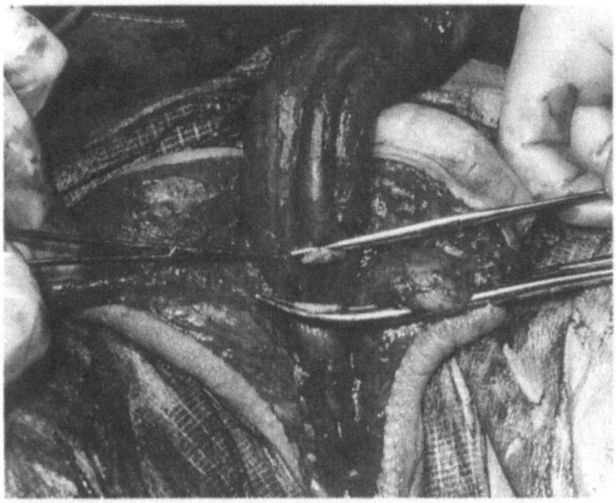

Fig. 3. Urethra and corpus spongiosum are cut after isolation from the corpora cavernosa

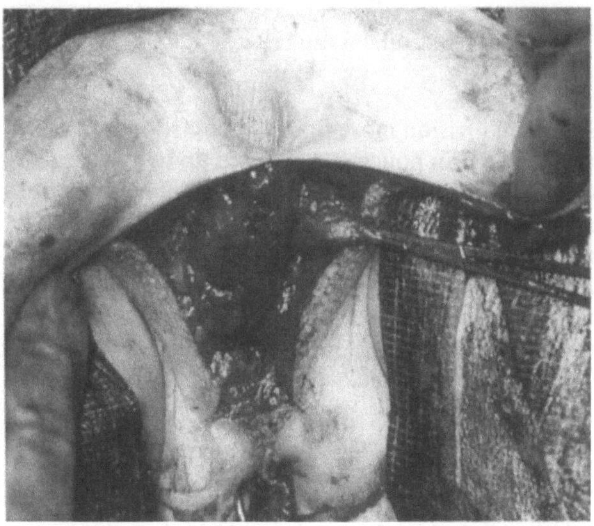

Fig. 4. The inverted penile skin pouch is brought into the cavity

the dissection can easily be done bluntly. Sometimes bundles of the levator ani have to be cut to give sufficient room. The metal probe in the urethra is now replaced by a catheter. The now inverted penile skin pouch is brought into the cavity by pulling on its pedicle (Fig. 4), and in the pedicle, the point is determined where the urethra is to be led out. A Y-shaped incision is made, and the urethra, together with its catheter, is pulled through this opening.

To facilitate the subsequent suturing of the urethra to the skin opening, I pass two stitches through the skin, fixing it on both sides of the urethra to the trigonum. The stitches can be removed at the end of the operation. Two stitches are led through the back edge of the inverted skin pouch close to each other, and the back of the skin pouch is incised in between these stitches. The stitches can now

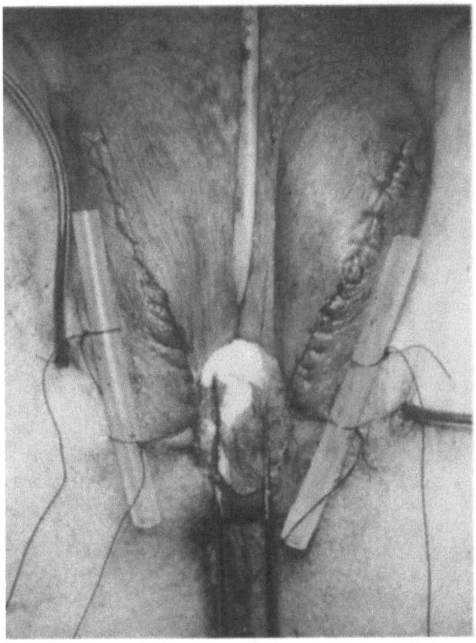

Fig. 5. The tampon in the vagina will be kept in place by retaining sutures. Both drains can be seen

be knotted to the end of the perineal incision more than 4–5 cm from each other. The defect in the posterior wall of the skin pouch can be filled up by the caudally pedicled perineal flap; this widens the introitus. The urethra is stitched to the skin opening, and the folds of scrotal skin on both sides are trimmed so that they get the shape of the labia majora. Two drains are left in place. To keep the inverted penile skin pouch in the cavity, a Vaseline-smeared tampon is used. To keep the tampon in the skin pouch, two stitches are led over the tampon through both labia and sutured on both sides over silicone tubes (Fig. 5). As my follow-up shows, this is a reliable technique, which gives few problems.

References

Edgerton MT, Bull J (1970) Surgical construction of the vagina and labia in male transsexuals. Plast Reconstr Surg 46:529

Jones HW Jr, Horst K, Schirmer A, Hoopes JE (1968) A sex conversion operation for males with transsexualism. Am J Obst Gynecol 95:101

Stuteville OH, Pandya NJ, Arieff AJ (1971) Surgical treatment of the male transsexual. In: Hueston JT (ed) Transactions of the Vth International Congress of Plastic and Reconstructive Surgery, Melbourne. Butterworth, London, p 1279

The Inverted Penis Skin Technique in Male-to-Female Transsexuals

W. Eicher

Frauenklinik, Diakonissenkrankenhaus, Mannheim, Akademisches Lehrkrankenhaus der Universität Heidelberg
Speyerer Str. 93, 6800 Mannheim 1, FRG

According to the present definition, transsexuals correspond in terms of their chromosomes, hormones, and anatomy to their phenotypic sexual characteristics but feel, with respect to their sexual identity, that they unmistakably belong to the opposite sex; For this reason, they wish to be reassigned to their psychological sex by means of endocrinological and surgical treatment. In genuine transsexuals the gender identity is irreversibly transposed and cannot be changed by any other therapy. They are convinced that they are living in the wrong body and do their utmost to have their genital organs transformed and their legal sexual status changed. The cause of this illness is unknown.

For the operation to take place, the diagnosis must have been made or confirmed by a specialist consultant. The final diagnostic report must be based on a period of consultation with the specialist which has lasted at least a year and must conclude that no other therapy is possible apart from endocrinological and surgical treatment, so that it would appear sensible to comply with the patient's wishes and adjust his sexual identity with the aim of achieving a stabilization of his personality. It has proved useful for the patient to have attempted beforehand – in the so-called real-life test – to live in the sexual role he wishes to adopt. This attempt should at least have been made during the phase of hormonal treatment. As a rule, following treatment with hormones of the opposite sex, gynecomasty and external feminization occur in male-to-female transsexuals. The hormonal treatment should be continuously administered for at least half a year prior to the operation and should be well tolerated, as hormonal substitution is necessary after the operation for the rest of the patient's life.

Technique

There are six basic stages of the transformation operation:

1. Castration by means of orchiectomy and resection of the spermatic cord
2. Formation of a cavity between urethra, bladder, peritoneum, and rectum
3. Stripping off the penis skin and amputation of the penis shaft
4. Invagination of the inverted penis skin
5. Creation of an orificium urethrae externum above the introitus neovaginae
6. Formation of a vulva, with large and small labia, and a clitoris.

Access is achieved via the perineum by means of a longitudinal incision in the raphe of scrotum. Both testicles are exposed and, after following the spermatic cord up to the anulus inguinalis superficialis, they are severed using clamps, with

Plastic Surgery in the Sexually Handicapped
Eds.: W. Eicher/Kubli/Herms

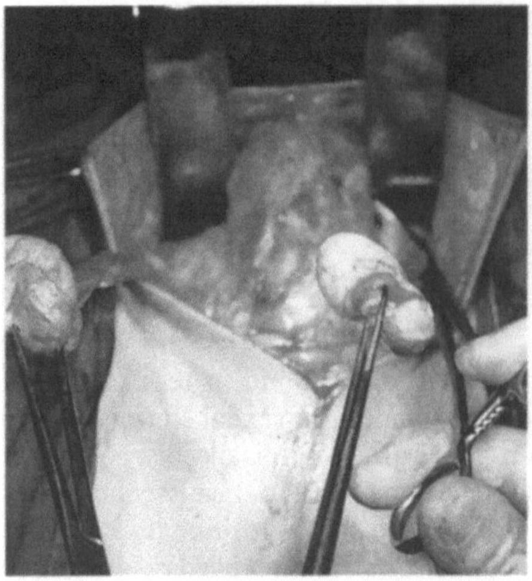

Fig. 1. Extirpation of the testicles using clamps, with ligations of spermatic cords

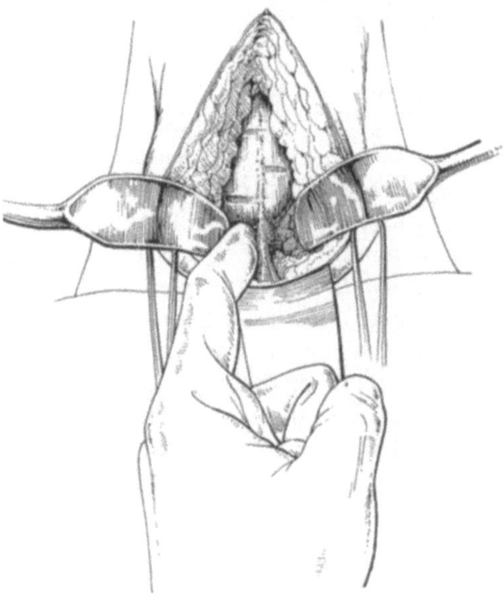

Fig. 2. To the side of the midline, the forefinger enters below the musculus transversus perinei superficialis and profundus into the loose tissue between rectum and urogenital apparatus

ligation of the spermatic cords (Fig. 1). The superficial perineal muscles are severed so that the midline of the tendinous center is seen. On this vertical line, the musculus bulbocavernosus is also attached. To the side of this midline, the forefinger can now enter carefully below the musculus transversus perinei superficialis and profundus into the loose tissue filling the space between rectum and urogenital apparatus, and it can penetrate through the fossa ischiorectalis to the prostate (Fig. 2). This is done on both sides of the midline. Then, Breisky specula are inserted, pushing the fibers of the levator ani muscle aside. Pronounced fibers of the pars prostatica of the levator muscle can be severed with scissors. Now, the tendinous centrum and its continuation, the musculus recto urethralis is cut through until the rear wall of the prostate and Denonvilliers' fascia is exposed

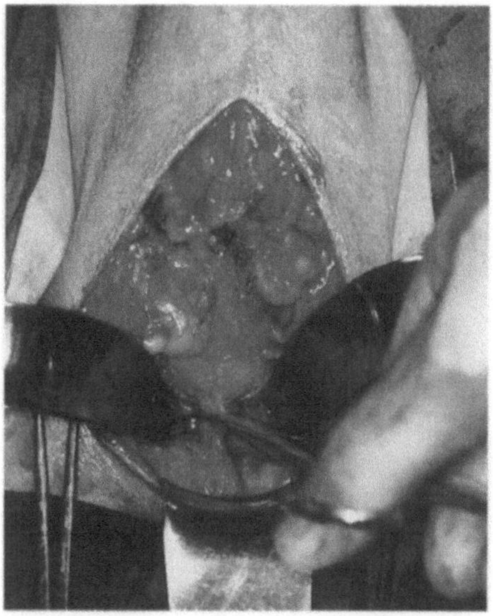

Fig. 3. Breisky specula pushing the levator muscles aside. Tendinous center and musculus rectourethralis are cut

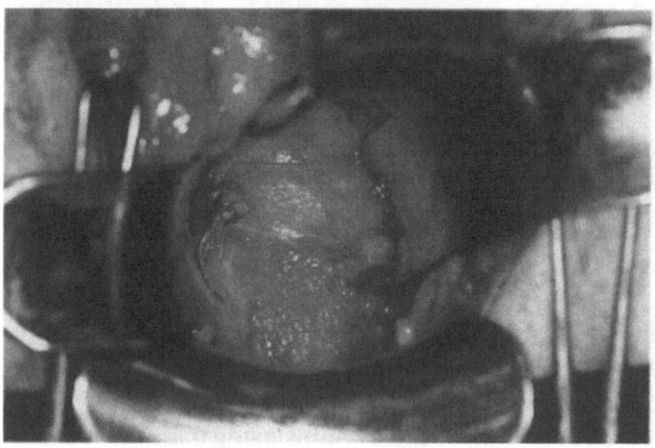

Fig. 4. Denovilliers' fascia is dissected, and rectum and bladder are separated up to the preperitoneal space

(Fig. 3). A broad incision is similarly made through the latter with the scissors. This has special importance with regard to providing the vagina with adequate depth. After the dissection of Denonvilliers' fascia, the rectum can be separated off obtusely up to the preperitoneal space. This results in an adequately large and deep cavity for the invagination of the penis skin (Fig. 4). Careful electrosurgical staunching of bleeding and ligation of spurting vessels is necessary, particularly in the area of the prostate rear wall and under the plexus surrounding the seminal vesicles. We swab the cavity thus formed with two gauze swabs.

After this, the penis shaft is stripped of its skin, the skin remaining attached at the mons pubis, its point of origin. The penis skin is severed at the corona glandis (Fig. 5). We do not implant the glans penis because this frequently leads to dis-

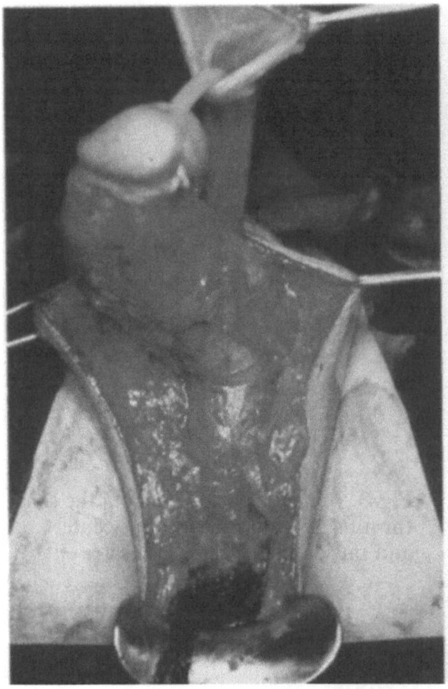

Fig. 5. Penis shaft is stripped of its skin, the skin remaining attached at the mons pubis and being severed at the corona glandis

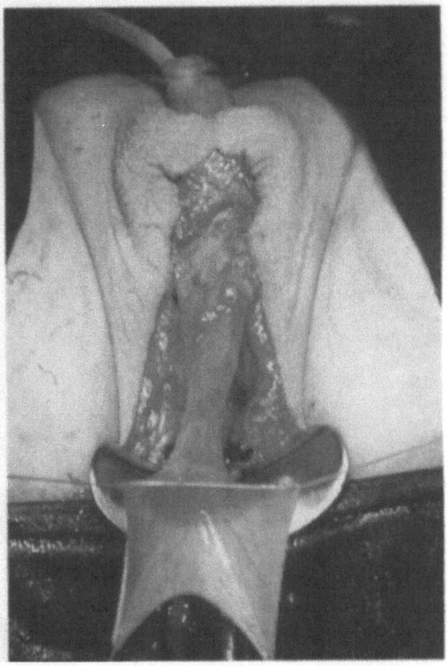

Fig. 6. The penis skin is inverted, and the urethra stump is led out under the symphysis through the inverted penis skin, which will now be invaginated, i.e., fixed in the preperitoneal space by Vicryl sutures

comfort and can cause complications. The musculus bulbocaveronsus and ischiocavernosus are cut away from the penis and resected; the urinary passage with the bulbus spongiosum is separated from the corpora cavernosa. After this, the spongy bodies can be removed on each side of the os pubis using clamps. We also resect the corpus spongiosum of the bulbus urethrae in order to prevent unpleasant swelling in the new vaginal introitus during the sexual reaction. Leaving spongy bodies, which some authors suggest, can lead to general discomfort; for this reason, we have had to perform corrective surgery in some transsexuals operated on elsewhere. The inverted penis skin can now be invaginated into the wound cavity prepared for the purpose. Prior to this, the urethra is led out through the inverted penis skin under the symphysis at the point where the orificium urethrae externum will later be formed (Fig. 6). The invaginated penis skin is now fixed in the preperitoneal space by means of four Vicryl sutures (Fig. 7). Before this, the cavity and the mons pubis are drained by means of a Redon drain tube, which emerges at the side of the perineum.

Now, the urethra is sutured to form an orificium externum below the symphysis in the female position (with 4×0 atraumatic catgut sutures). By resecting scrotal skin and pulling down two lateral cusps of skin, large and small labia are simu-

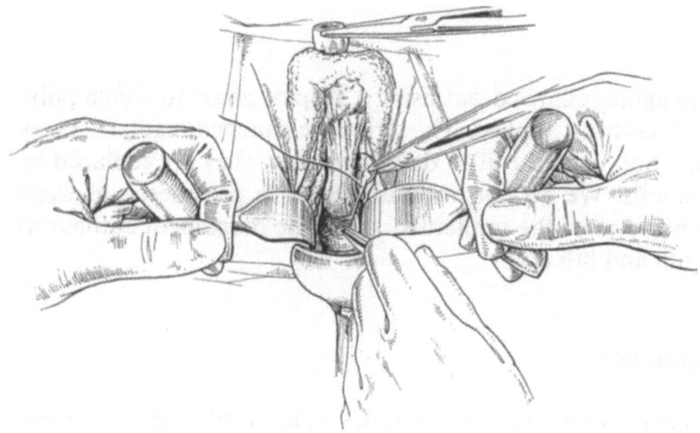

Fig. 7. Inverted penis skin is fixed in the preperitoneal space by Vicryl sutures

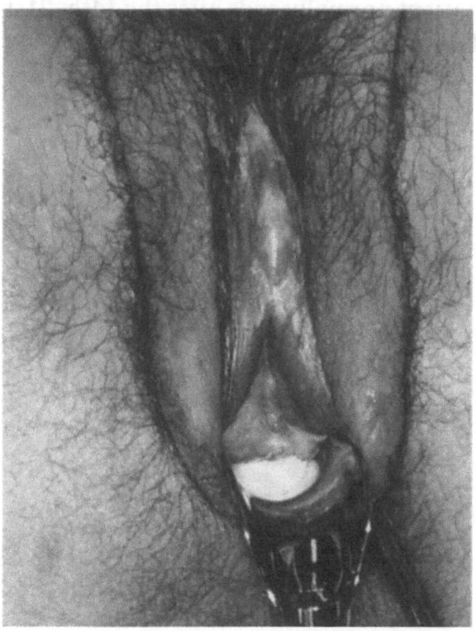

Fig. 8. By resecting scrotal skin and pulling down two lateral cusps of skin, large and small labia are simulated. A piece of cutaneous spongy body tissue removed from the glans penis is freely transplanted as a pseudoclitoris

lated. The rear circumference of the inverted penis skin is stitched to the perineal skin. A clitoris-like ridge over the urethra is created by means of suitable take-up stitching with Prolene, which is removed on the 12th day after the operation. A piece of cutaneous spongy body tissue the size of a pumpkin seed, previously removed from the glans penis, is freely transplanted over this ridge. To this end, an area of the same size must first be disepithelized (Fig. 8). The stitches in the skin are formed using non reabsorbable Prolene threads, which are removed on or about the 10th day.

Postoperative Care

Tamponage of the neovagina is carried out using a strip of gauze to which polyvidone-iodine ointment has been applied. The strips are changed regularly every 2–4 days after the operation until the 10th day; thereafter, they are replaced by a silicone rubber prosthesis. We do not normally use firm prostheses, as these would cause pressure necrosis of the implanted skin. The permanent catheter is removed between the 6th and 8th day.

Complications and Outcome

The implanted penis skin does not always take completely. In 50% of cases, there is only a partial take. However, generally speaking, epithelization sets in quickly, as there is only partial necrosis. Adequate bouginage, which holds the neovagina open, is important; otherwise, particularly in the case of partial necrosis, some shrinkage may occur. Treatment as an inpatient normally ends after the 14th–21st day. There is only a slight tendency for the vaginoid to shrink; however, for only minor shrinkage to occur, there must be regular bouginage until the commence-

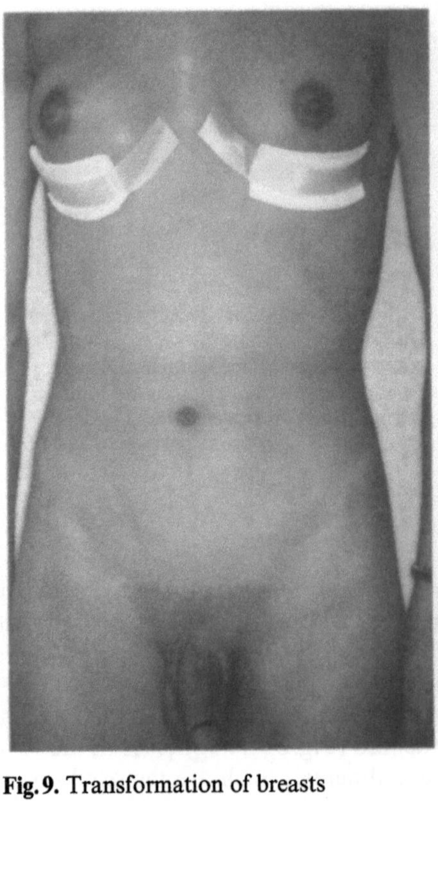

Fig. 9. Transformation of breasts

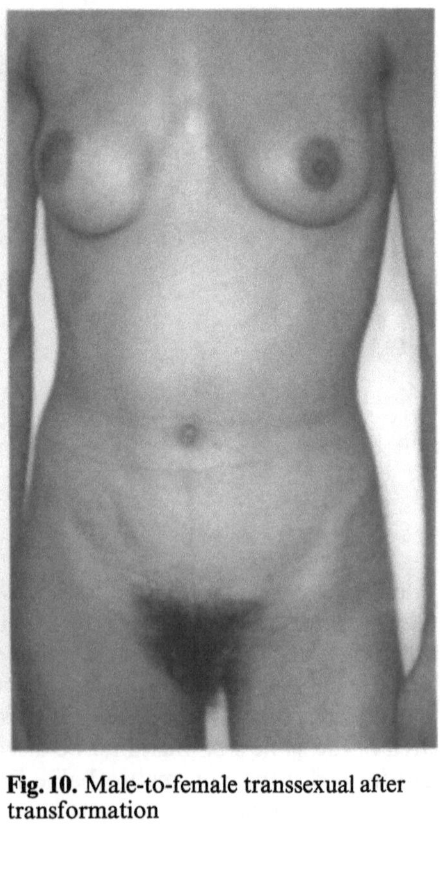

Fig. 10. Male-to-female transsexual after transformation

ment of regular sexual intercourse. For this purpose, in addition to the prosthesis given to the patient, the use of a vibrator has proved effective. Stenoses and shortening of the vagina have been observed in 15% of cases. An unpleasant complication, which we have observed three times recently, is the papillomavirus infection, with an extended lawn of condylomata accompanying inflammation and shrinkage of the vaginoid.

Stenosis at the orificium urethrae externum is relatively rare (5%) and hardly occurs at all if the spongy body around the bulbus urethrae is removed. It is important that the urethra is not resected in a circular, but in an oval form. Urethral stenoses can be succesfully treated by bouginage using Hegar obturators (without narcosis). A urinary fistula has never occurred with the technique practised by us. The likelihood of a rectovaginal fistula is 1%. It is important to notice any damage to, or perforation of, the rectum and to repair it. As a rule, this makes it possible to prevent fistulae. We were able to close the two rectovaginal fistulae with which we have hitherto been confronted without colostomy.

For more than a year, we have regularly been putting antibiotic prophylactic measures into practice, using piperacillin (Pipril). In addition, we put the patients on a so-called astronauts' diet for a week to prevent defecation in this time; this fosters better hygiene conditions and promotes the healing process. Mammatransformation results form hormonal treatment causing gynecomastia. If the increase is regarded as not sufficient, augmentation can be achieved by implanting inflatable mammaprothesis (Figs. 9, 10). To date, we have performed more than 200 such operations. None of the patients has regretted having undergone surgery.

Reference

Eicher W (1984) Transsexualismus. Möglichkeiten und Grenzen der Geschlechtsumwandlung (Transsexualität, Possibilities and Limits of Sexual Transformation).

Rectosigmoid Vaginoplasty

D. R. Laub[1] and D. R. Laub[2] II

[1] Gender Dysphoria Program, Inc., 900 Welch Road, Suite 402,
Palo Alto, CA 94304, USA
[2] Medical College of Wisconsin, 8701 Watertown Plank Road Milwaukee, Wisconsin, USA

The purpose of this contribution is to describe the use of rectosigmoid for vaginal construction, the advantage being that it is more natural and yet is associated with a surprisingly low complication rate. We have used the technique for vaginal agenesis, testicular feminization syndrome, and gender dysphoria in a total of 45 cases. This experience follows experience with 170 cases of vaginal construction using the classical McIndoe thick split-thickness skin graft technique. The technique of sigmoid vaginostomy used in Russia (Alexandrov 1955) and Eastern Europe in more than 700 cases may be similar in many ways (Kunz 1975).

This technique utilizes a 15-cm segment of upper rectum and lower sigmoid colon for construction of the upper two-thirds to three-quarters of the vagina. The use of other portions of the intestine for the vagina is not new, having been described years ago (Pratt 1961); in fact, the Baldwin technique described in 1904 predates most of the various other methods of vaginal construction now extant.

Some advantages of the use of rectosigmoid are apparent; others are not as obvious:

1. Sensibility is retained in this colonic segment.
2. Natural lubrication is present, without excessive mucus production (Golligher 1986).
3. Vigorous arterial supply is maintained.
4. The malodor associated with skin placed in a body cavity is not present.
5. Long-term use of a stent is not necessary.
6. Skin graft donor site scar is absent.
7. Examination reveals normal tactile feeling and visual qualities.
8. Squamous cell cancer has been reported in skin vaginas (Abrenio 1977; Imrie et al. 1986; Rotmensch 1983; Steffanof 1973).

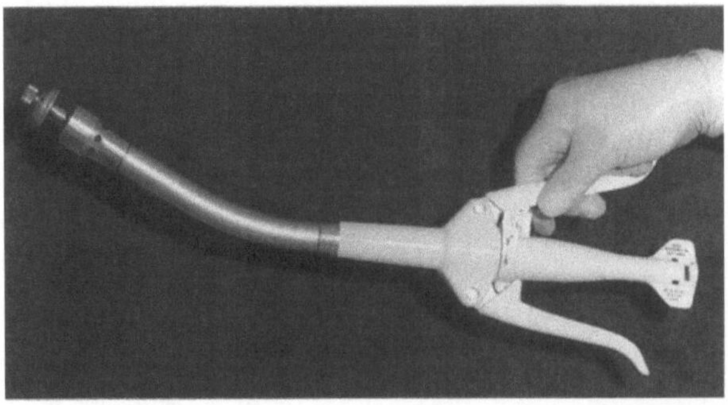

Fig. 1. The stapling device used for rectosigmoid vaginoplasty

Plastic Surgery in the Sexually Handicapped
Eds.: W. Eicher/Kubli/Herms

A technological breakthrough from Russia helped make this technique safer: the stapling device (Fig. 1). In years past, prior to the introduction of the intestinal stapler (Cohn and Nance 1986), the rate of leaks from low anterior resection, i.e., anastomosis below the peritoneal reflection, was 25% (Cohn and Nance 1986), but with the use of the stapling device the leak rate is only 1%–3% (Ravitch and Steichen 1979). Conditions are optimized (R. H. Lee and M. Trollope, personal communication), and the complication rate is minimized, when the surgery is performed (a) by a highly experienced and technically expert surgeon; (b) upon relatively young, healthy patients; and (c) with the end-to-end anastomosis (EEA) stapler positioned via the anus for coloniç anastomosis.

We originally gained experience using intestine 14 years ago: the sigmoid rather than the rectosigmoid was used as an island vascular flap to provide fresh tissue for the repair of postoperative rectovaginal fistula following vaginal reconstruction in gender dysphoria patients. This technique had been described by Markland (1974) a urologic surgeon of the University of Minnesota and later Louisiana State University. The anastomosis was made above the peritoneal reflection, reanastomosis to achieve bowel continuity was accomplished with sutures, and viability was supported by little more than the marginal artery of Drummond. The technique was generally successful, but the bowel was not vigorous and robust with respect to its blood supply.

Technique

A modified lithotomy position allows two teams to work simultaneously, thus significantly reducing the time of operating. A low transverse abdominal incision and perineal incisions are employed. The perineal dissection opens a cavity up to the peritoneum, while from above, a 15 cm segment (Fig. 2) of intestine is located and surgically isolated. This segment is based on the unpaired superior hemorrhoidal artery system from the inferior mesenteric, which is from the aorta itself (Fig. 3). The segment is taken out of the gastrointestinal stream and only moved about 7.5 cm to its new vaginal position (Fig. 4). Little mesentery and little vascular and nerve suply is disturbed. Continuity is reestablished using the EEA sta-

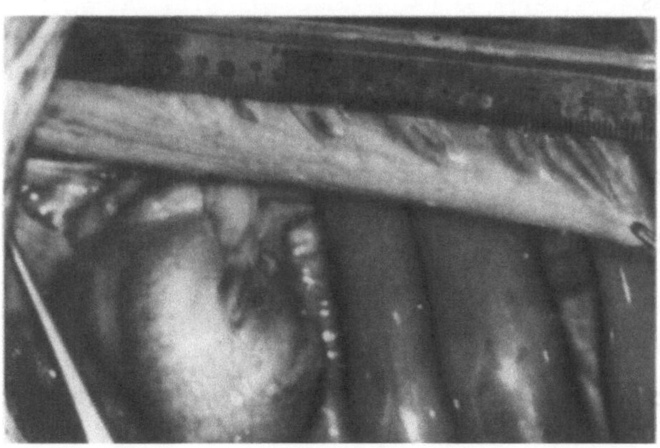

Fig. 2. A segment of intestine 15 cm in length is isolated from the peritoneal reflection upward. Nerve and blood supply is virtually undisturbed

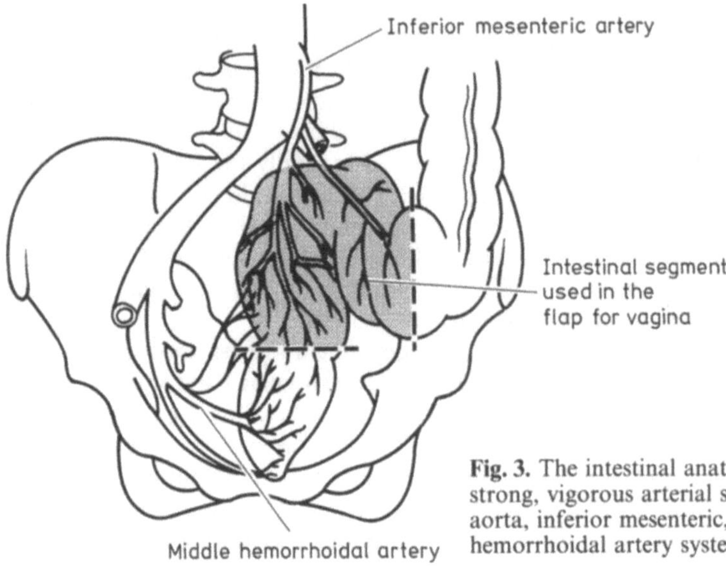

Fig. 3. The intestinal anatomy and the strong, vigorous arterial supply from the aorta, inferior mesenteric, and superior hemorrhoidal artery system

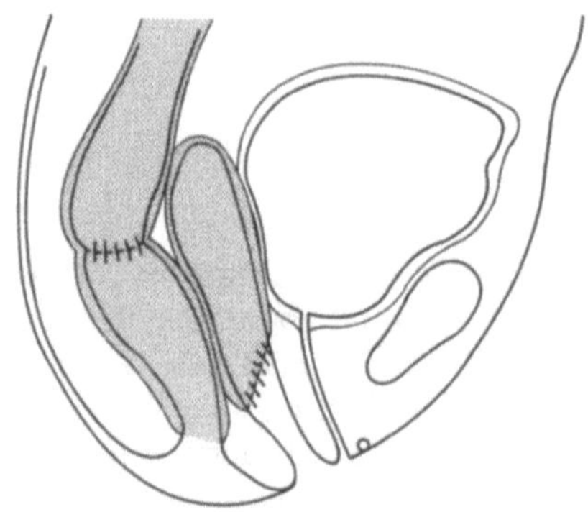

Fig. 4. Position of the new vagina and the suture line. The segment usually does not come all the way down to the perineum; flaps of skin are usually necessary to form the lower vagina segment

pling machine (Fig. 1), positioned via the anus. Because this intestinal flap does not reach the perineum (Fig. 4), skin flaps are necessary from adjacent labia, perineum, groin, or scrotal areas.

A stent is used intermittently for 6 weeks to 6 months, a frequency of twice per day being adequate. A pneumatic inflatable stent (Heyer-Schulte, Mentor Corp., Goleta, California) is used for 10 days, then a silicone foam stent covered with a latex rubber condom (Precision Ocular Prosthetics, Redwood City, California). Fashioning a longer colon circumference with darts, Z-plasty, and/or a bias cut decreases the incidence of circumferential contracture at the colon-skin anastomosis. Douching only produces excess mucus production.

Anatomy

The important clinical aspect of the anatomy is that we use the colon at the level of the peritoneal reflection(or a little below), at a point where the inferior mesenteric artery and vein, and the sympathetic and parasympathetic mesenteric nerve distribution systems, are merging with another system: the middle rectal (hemorrhoidal) artery, vein, and nerves. The middle rectal system is also accompanied by sympathetic and parasympathetic nerves. There is no significant interruption of arteries (Fig. 3), veins, or nerves to the remaining distal or proximal portions of intestine when this site of disconnection is selected. Neither does transfer of the intestine to the new vaginal position require vascular or nerve interruption. Thus, the rectal stump has excellent middle hemorrhoidal blood supply, and the transferred colon has excellent inferior mesenteric/superior hemorrhoidal supply. From an anatomic point of view, this site of disconnection is logical (Fig. 4).

Innervation is from the autonomic system, with sympathetic and parasympathetic components. The nerves follow the path of the blood supply closely. The sympathetics, which are primarily vasomotor in function, arise as preganglionic fibers in the first three lumbar segments of the spinal cord. They synapse in the ganglionic sympathetic chains on either side and emerge as lumbar splanchnic nerves. They join the preaortic plexus, and fibers from both the thoracic splanchnic nerves and celiac plexus, and are distributed as the inferior mesenteric plexus, accompanying the inferior mesenteric artery and vein. These fibers do not follow the smaller blood vessels, but proceed directly to all the pelvic organs supplied.

The parasympathetic nervi erigentes are derived from the sacral autonomics, which spring from the second, third, and fourth sacral nerves. These have been shown to travel upwards to the inferior mesenteric plexus and be distributed along the course of the inferior mesenteric artery.

The ability of the brain to perceive vibration and pleasure, and to differentiate gas from liquid and from solid, may be facilitated by these nerve pathways.

Physiology

The large intestine receives ileal contents, absorbs water and electrolytes, and acts as a reservoir for feces. It is insensitive to stimuli which would produce pain if applied to skin, but it is sensitive to distension; however, a great difference exists between the colonic and the rectal appreciation of this stimulus. In the rectum, detection of small amounts of flatus and differentiation between gas, liquid, and solid feces is possible (Goligher 1975). A good appreciation of vibratory stimuli is present in the transferred rectosigmoids of our patients.

Protective mucus is secreted throughout the bowel by the columnar cells known as goblet cells. Any irritation of the mucous membrane produces a discharge of mucus by the goblet cells. There is no evidence of nervous or humoral control of the release of mucus by these cells; it is a local phenomenon. The rectum has been found by some workers to absorb no water, or to absorb less than the higher portions of the large intestine (Goligher 1975). At any rate, use of the 15 cm rectosigmoid segment does not interrupt colonic physiology with respect to absorption, mucus production, or sensibility, and it does not produce diarrhea for more than a few days. Excess mucus production, compared with vaginal standards, is less of a problem than when other segments of the gastrointestinal tract are used (Goligher 1983).

Results

Our experience with 45 operations shows that the technique has evolved. The first seven operations used the intestinal tract, but not the stapling device and not low sigmoid/upper rectum. Subsequently, we used the lower segments and the new stapling device in a series of 33 operations. In this latter series, there have been no complications other than minor stenosis at the skin-to-intestine circumferential suture line and one early obstruction at the suture line, treated by dilation. This problem is precluded by early dilation, more viable skin flaps, and particularly a bias cut on the colon or a dart cut type of Z-plasty to increase the circumferential length of the intestine.

Of particular note, there has been 0% incidence of anastomosis leak or vascular death of the transplant. All patients report some sensibility and success with sexual intercourse when attempted. With colonoscopy the appearance seems rather normal. With digital examination, the characteristics of smoothness and lubrication are appreciated to a supranormal degree (Fig. 5).

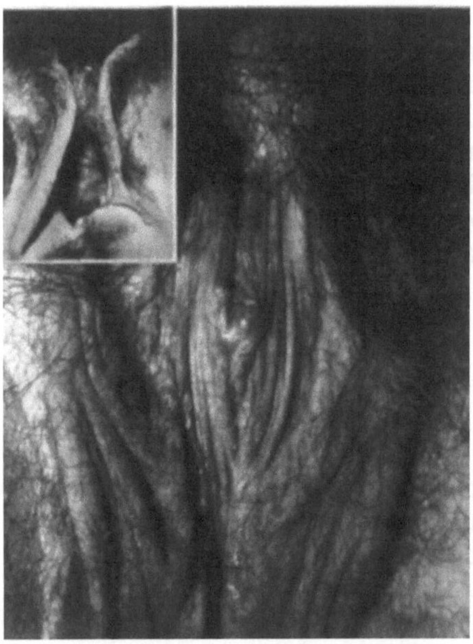

Fig. 5. Results of rectosigmoid vaginoplasty. The *inset* shows sexual climax in the postoperative transsexual

Discussion

Use of other segments of intestine requires an island pedicle technique, which involves removal of nerve supply and partial devascularization, occasionally to the point of marginal blood supply. Disadvantages to use of the ileum include (a) bleeding with coital trauma to the thin mucosa, (b) excessive mucus secretion, (c) periumbilical pain with intercourse, and (d) tendency to prolapse. This transfer of rectosigmoid involves no significant removal of nerve or blood supply. Furthermore, the upper rectum contains sensory nerve supply sufficiently discerning to differentiate between gas, liquid, and solid stool, and nerves to notify the cerebrum when the rectum is distended.

Lubrication. Natural lubrication is not available to postoperative patients with skin flaps or grafts, and at the other end of the spectrum, excessive mucus production has been known to follow transfer of ileum. The transferred rectosigmoid, however, has natural lubrication without soiling, unless excessively stimulated. Another reason for continence of mucus might be that in this technique the distal vagina is constructed from skin flaps. Furthermore, the distal sigmoid and rectum absorbs more fluid than it secretes.

Examination of these rectosigmoid-derived vaginas similar to the postoperative examination of our previous 180 vaginal reconstructions (utilizing skin only) revealed a more natural presentation from both a tactile and a visual standpoint. The perception is that there is "no friction at all" on the surface of this new tissue.

Safety and Complications. The disadvantages of this technique are that the operation is a more major one, the abdominal cavity is entered, and the gastrointestinal tract is opened (Table 1). The time of surgery is not prolonged because two teams operate simultaneously.

The general surgery team involved in our cases has used the stapler in more than 260 cases of bowel anastomosis, with (amazingly) only 2 minor self-healing leaks, 1 requiring a colostomy. No leaks occurred in any of the cases reported in this series (R. H. Lee and M. Trollope, personal communication).

Table 1. Advantages and disadvantages of rectosigmoid versus skin for vaginoplasty

	Rectosigmoid	Skin
Advantages	More natural No stent necessary No contraction No donor scar Less secondary surgery Less bed rest Lubrication Some sensibility More success in obtaining a functional vagina	More minor surgery Does not enter abdominal cavity
Disadvantages	Enters abdominal cavity (6 weeks convalescence) Possible complications Anastomotic leak (peritonitis) Later intestinal obstruction Vascular death of the pedicle graft 9-day vs 7-day hospitalization Abdominal scar	Donor site scar Stent necessary Contraction Immobilization for 7 days Odor Lubrication necessary Some size problems

AIDS. The acquired immune deficiency syndrome (AIDS) virus has been said to be transmitted across the rectal mucosa in the manner of transfer of venereal disease. The thought has occurred that the rectosigmoid vagina would be a site of AIDS virus transfer, more so than a genetic vagina, but this has not been the case.

Selection Criteria for Gender Dysphoria Patients. The gender dysphoria patients have been referred by the Gender Dysphoria Program of Palo Alto, Inc. [California Foundation (501.C.3) set up in 1980 to assist patients with gender dysphoria syndrome, and to carry out public education in this area]. The criteria for selection of patients with gender dysphoria syndrome are more stringent than the minimal standards of the Harry Benjamin Gender Dysphoria Association, the international professional association which has set down guidelines for surgical selection, accepted by the medical and legal professions, and the insurance industry.

The patient must be recommended for the surgery by two behavioral scientists, in writing. One of these must have known the patient in a professional psychotherapeutic relationship for 6 months. The patient must have been completely and succesfully living in the genetically opposite sex role for at least 1 year – passing the so-called real-life test. Prior to the surgical gender reassignment, the patient must have accomplished hormonal sex reassignment, which is of both diagnostic and therapeutic value. Hormonal treatment requires physical examination, and liver and blood chemistries measured yearly. In their recommendation, the two advocates must inform the surgeon not only that the 1 year of cross-living has been successful, but that the essential diagnostic features of the condition have been present continuously for 2 years or more, i.e., demonstration of discomfort in the gender role, the urge to rid the self of genitalia, freedom from psychosis, and the intense desire to change.

Summary

The technique of vaginal construction utilizing rectosigmoid is made possible by the EEA stapling device, originally developed in Europe and coming into more widespread use in North America in the last 10 years. The technique is applied to both vaginal atresia and gender dysphoria patients. A low complication rate is noted, and patients enjoy the advantages of a more natural substitution for an absent vagina.

References

Abrenio JK, Chung HI, Pomante R (1977) Verrucous CA arising from an artificial vagina. Obstet Gynecol 50:185–215

Alexandrov MS (1955) Obrazovanie iskustvennogo ulagalishcha iz sigmoidnoi kishki (Formation of an artificial vagina from sigmoid colon). Mediz, Moscow

Baldwin JF (1904) The formation of an artificial vagina by intestinal transplantation. Ann Surg 40:398–403

Cohn I, Nance FC (1986) The colon and rectum: anatomy and surgical procedures. In: Sabiston DC Jr (ed) Textbook of surgery: the Biologic Basis for Modern Surgical Practice, 13th edn. Saunders, Philadelphia, pp 983–987

Duckler L (1972) Squamous cell carcinoma developing in an artificial vagina. Obstet Gynecol 40:35

Goligher JC (1975) Surgery of the anus, rectum and colon, 3rd edn. Baillière Tindall, London

Goligher JC (1983) The use of pedicled transplants of sigmoid and other parts of the intestine for vaginal constructions. Ann R Coll Surg Eng 65:353–355

Imrie JEA, Kennedy JH, Holmes JD, McGrouther DH (1986) Intraepithelial neoplasia arising in an artificial vagina. Br J Obstet Gynecol 93:886–889

Kalinina TV, Kasulin VS (1966) Apparat KTs-28 dlia sshivaniia priamoi kishki s tolstoi ili tonkoi kishkoi (Apparatus „KC-28“ for suturing the rectum to the colon or small intestine). Vopr Onkol 12:114–118

Laub DR, Fisk N (1974) A rehabilitation program for gender dysphoria syndrome by surgical sex change. Plast Reconstr Surg 53:388

Markland C (1974) Use of the colon in treating complications of transexual surgery. Paper presented at VII Interdisciplinary Symposium of the Harry Benjamin International Gender Dysphoria Association, Stanford, 1974

Pratt JH (1961) Sigmoidovaginostomy: a new method of obtaining satisfactory vaginal depth. Am J Obstet Gynecol 81:535–545

Ravitch NM, Steichen FM (1979) A stapling instrument for end-to-end inverting anastomoses of the gastrointestinal tract. Ann Surg 189:791–797

Shirodkar VN, Rotmensch J, Rosenhein N, Dillon M, Murphy A, Woodruff J (1983) Carcinoma arising in the neovagina: a case report and review of the literature. Obstet Gynecol 61:534–536

Steffanof DN (1973) Late development of squamous carcinoma in a split skin graft lining the vagina. Plast Reconstr Surg 51:454–456

Surgical Treatment of Female-to-Male Transsexuals

W. Eicher

Frauenklinik, Diakonissenkrankenhaus, Mannheim, Akademisches Lehrkrankenhaus der Universität Heidelberg,
Speyerer Strasse 93, 6800 Mannheim, FRG

Like their male-to-female counterparts, female-to-male transsexuals have a permanently and irreversibly transposed gender identity. Basically, these patients totally lack any motivation to change their gender consciousness, which is why psychotherapy directed toward this end cannot be successful. The patients are convinced that they are living in the wrong body and do their utmost to have their genital organs transformed and their sexual status changed. The transformation does not involve a change of sex, but constitutes an adjustment of the body to the psychological gender. Hormone treatment and the operation create the necessary preconditions for psychological stabilization.

Endocrinological-surgical therapy may only be commenced when the diagnosis has been made or confirmed by a specialist consultant. The period of consultation must amount to a minimum of 1 year. After this time, the specialist concludes that it would appear sensible to comply with the patient's wish to undergo endocrinological and surgical adjustment to bring bodily features into line with the psychological gender identity since the latter cannot be changed by psychotherapy.

As in the case of male-to-female transsexuals, with female-to-male transsexuals there is a rule that the patient must be treated with hormones of the opposite sex for at least half a year prior to the operation. Thereafter, the hormone substitution therapy must be continued for the rest of the patient's life. In the case of female-to-male transsexuals, the result is a distinct development of masculine features, with breaking of the voice and growth of beard.

We perform the genital transformation operation on female-to-male transsexuals in three stages: (a) the vaginal colpohysterectomy, with extirpation of the adnexa uteri; (b) the operation to transform the female breasts; and (c) the formation of the clitoris penoid with surrogate testicles.

Vaginal Colpohysterectomy with Extirpation of Adnexa Uteri

The extirpation of the uterus with the adnexa is normally carried out successfully and without particular difficulty – even in the case of nulliparas – by an experienced surgeon through the vagina (Fig. 1). Even a leiomyoma uteri of fist size can be removed, by morcellation, from the body of a woman who has not yet borne any children. Extended access through the vagina is possible by means of a lateral Schuchardt's incision. However, this is normally unnecessary: a small longitudinal incision in the posterior commissure suffices.

Plastic Surgery in the Sexually Handicapped
Eds.: W. Eicher/Kubli/Herms

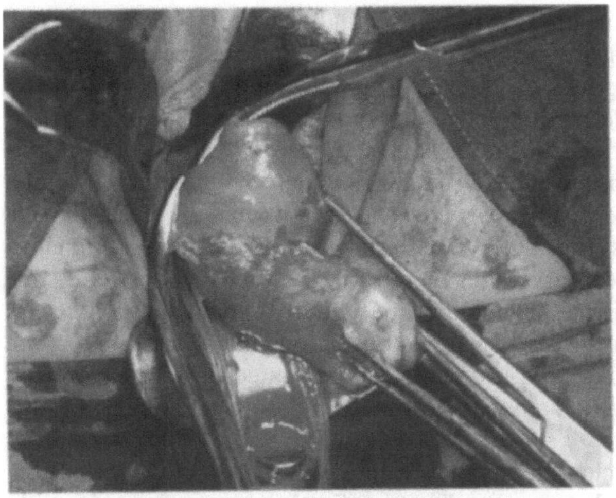

Fig. 1. Extirpation of the uterus through the vagina

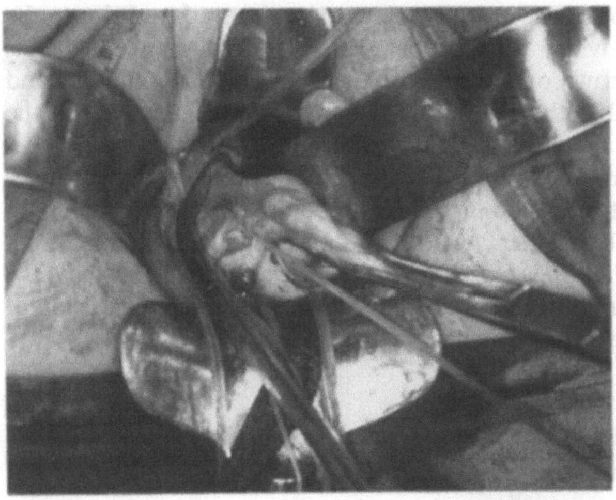

Fig. 2. Extirpation of the adnexa (ovaries and tubes) through the vagina

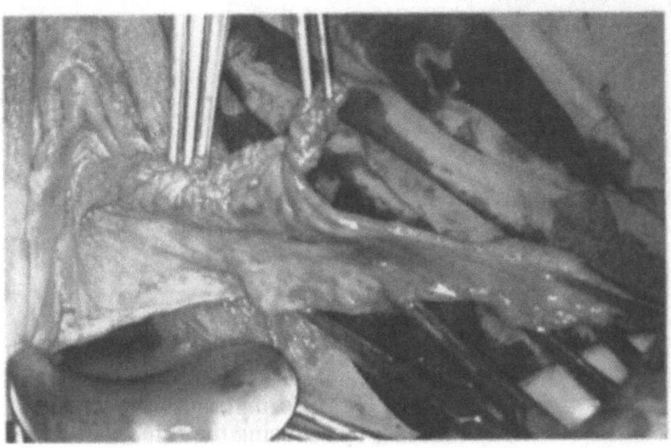

Fig. 3. Extirpation of the vagina

After disinfection of the vagina, the portio vaginalis cervicis is hooked up and pulled forward. After cutting around the cervix, the bladder and rectum are separated from the uterus. The pouch of Douglas is opened, and the sacrouterine ligaments and uterine bundle of vessels are severed by means of clamps. After opening the plica vesicouterina, the uterus is turned over and cut away from the adnexa and the ligamentum teres uteri. The adnexa can be pulled forward, and the ligamenta infundibulo pelvica ligated. The ovaries and tubes are resected from their remaining connections (Fig. 2). Extraperitonization of the stumps and closure of the peritoneum with catgut sutures then follow.

From a longitudinal incision through the front and rear vaginal walls, the vaginal skin is separated from the bladder fascia on the one hand, and the rectum towards the side, on the other, and is completely extirpated up to the introitus (Fig. 3). There follows a careful staunching of bleeding, both electrically and by stitching.

The wound cavity is not closed permanently in order to prevent the formation of abscesses, hematomas, and empyemas. First, we firmly tampon the cavity with a strip of gauze. The perineum is built up considerably by means of sutures of the musculus levator and bulbocavernosus to a point below the urethra. Prior to the operation, the patient is provided with a suprapubic bladder drainage, which is removed after the strip is drawn out. We loosen the tampon on the 2nd day and remove it gradually up to the 6th day. Within the next 4 weeks, the walls of the cavity adhere to each other up to the vaginal entrance below the urethra.

In the first 10 days after removal of the strip, careful spreading with a finger is carried out so that the introitus does not close up before the sides of the upper part of the cavity have stuck together. As a rule, a small indentation remains below the urethra. This indentation is closed up in the course of the next step – the displacement of the urethra up to the tip of the clitoris after disepithelization of the former by taking up the muscle stitches.

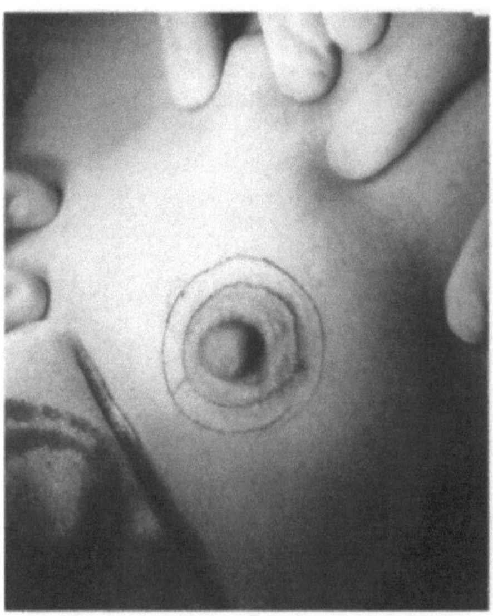

Fig. 4. Transformation of the female breast by reducing the skin

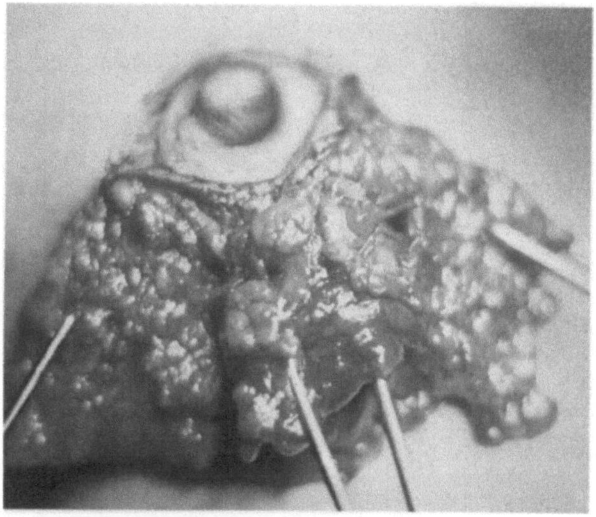

Fig. 5. Transformation of the female breast by subcutaneous mastectomy

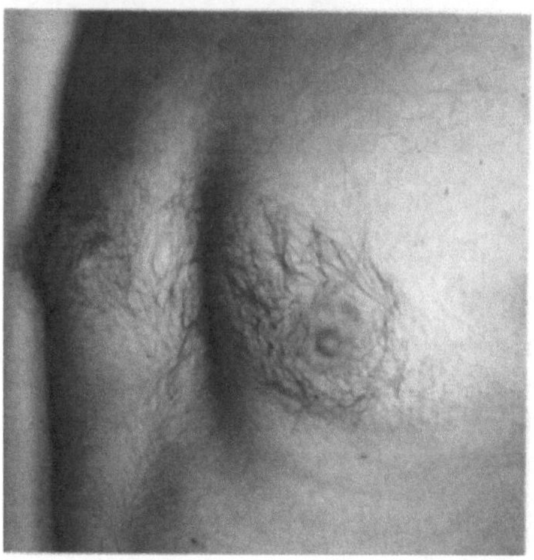

Fig. 6. Breast after surgical transformation and androgen therapy

Transformation of Female Breast

If the female breast is small, it is reduced in size by a subcutaneous mastectomy, with periareolar reduction of skin (Figs. 4–6). In the case of large breasts, ablatio mammae is carried out, with free retransplantation of the reduced-size mamilla.

Clitoris Penoid with Surrogate Testicles

As a result of androgen therapy, there is normally a slight hypertrophy of the clitoris. The clitoris can be displaced by a reverse Y-incision on the mons veneris, and the urinary passage can be extended to the tip of the clitoris, after refreshing

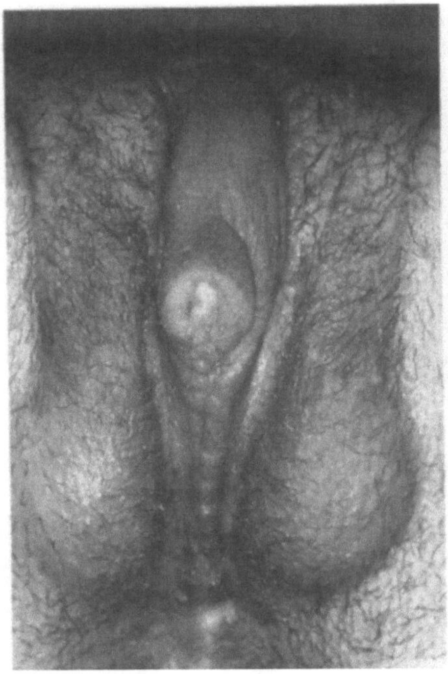

Fig. 7. Clitoris penoid with surrogate testicles. The urinary passage is extended to the tip of the clitoris

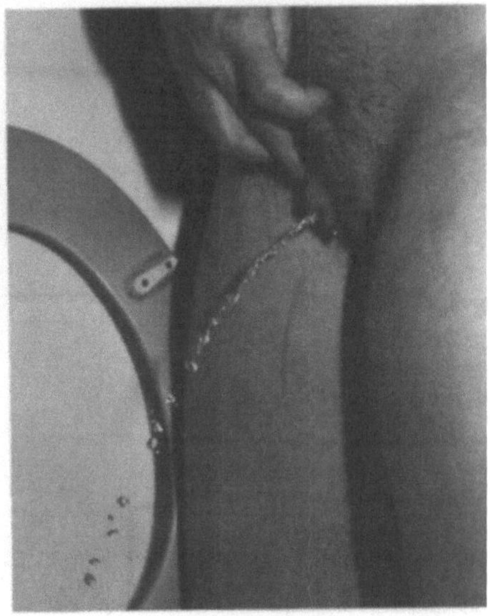

Fig. 8. Extension of the urinary passage to the tip of the clitoris enables the patient to urinate in a standing position

and partial resection of the small labia. Prior to this, a suburethral sinus must be disepithelized and closed by taking up lateral tissue and the musculus bulbocavernosus. The first layer of the refreshed labia above the catheter that opens out at the tip of the clitoris is laid over the catheter tension-free, using 4 × 0 atraumatic catgut sutures. A second row of stitches is put in on the outside of the freshened labia, using Prolene thread, which is removed on the 10th day.

After the displacement of the clitoris and before surgery on the urinary passage, two Silastic implants, for wich two pockets have previously been prepared, are inserted in what were originally the large labia. The final result is shown in Fig. 7.

The operation has achieved its purpose if the patient can urinate in a standing position; for the patient, this is an important feature of masculinity (Fig. 8).

Abdominal Tubular Pedicle Flap Penoid

The abdominal tubular pedicle flap penoid is no longer recommended by us, as the functional results are not usually satisfactory. The technique is described elsewhere (Eicher 1984 and Laub et al. in this book). A penoid is formed from a diagonal tubular pedicle flap. It is either initially stiffened or slowly, in several

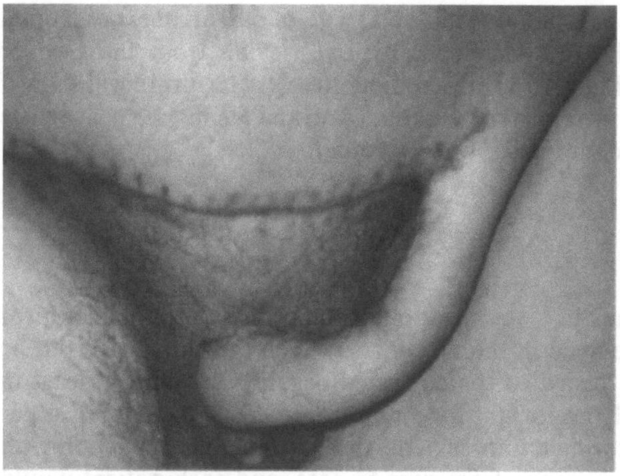

Fig. 9. The abdominal tubular pedicle flap penoid which is relocated in several stages to its position under the mons pubis

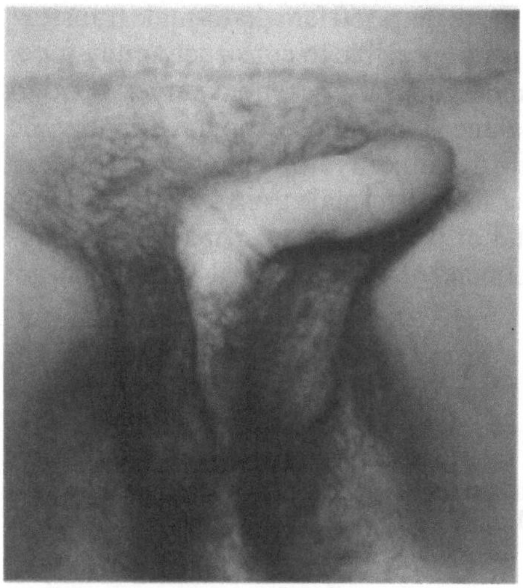

Fig. 10. The abdominal tubular flap penoid shown in Fig. 9

stagees, provided with a urethre to wards the tip. Finally, surrogate testicles can be implanted in the large labia (Fig. 9, 10).

We initially constructed a passage for the subsequent urethra horizontally and only then formed the final tubular pedicle flap. We relocated this flap in several stages to the right position under the mons pubis, and finally stiffened it by means of a silicone prosthesis. However, this is a very time-consuming procedure: in the case in question, a total of 15 inpatient operations were necessary, in part because of fistulas alongside the urethra which had to be closed in several steps.

We have followed up 10 abdominally tubular pedicle flapped phalluses operated on by a urologist department in Munich. In only two cases intravaginal coitus was possible and the phallus was insensitive. There were either problems with stiffening protheses or with the urethra.

We consider the flap techniques for phalloplasty to be still at an experimental stage and are observing the results refered by Laub et al. from the Gender Dysphoria Program Inc. in Palo Alto with a major interest. The future will show if the postmodern phalloplasties reported by Laub, Laub and Hentz (see next article in this book) will be the technological breakthrough.

Results and Satisfaction

As a rule, the operation leads to a stabilization of the personality, to a compromise which allows life to be lived in the sexual role which the patient feels to be his. The local results with regard to the corrected organs vary and, at least in many cases, are not crucially important for an improvement in the overall situation. In the case of female-to-male transsexuals, there is general satisfaction with the operations, which vary in scope from case to case, and each patient would again wish to have his physical sexual features adjusted by surgery under the same circumstances. We have now operated on more than 150 female-to-male transsexuals. All patients were clearly told that it is not possible to construct a fully functional penis. The patients who have not undergone clitorispenoid surgery tend to be psychologically more stable and well balanced than those who have undergone repeated multiple corrective surgery with the objective of obtaining a tubular pedicle flap phallus. It is notable that most female-to-male transsexuals maintain very stable partnerships and live in marital or permanent, near-marital relationships after hormonal and surgical adjustment of their physical sexual characteristics.

Reference

Eicher W (1984) Transsexualismus, Möglichkeiten und Grenzen der Geschlechtsumwandlung (Transsexualism, Possibilities and Limits of Sexual Transformation). Fischer, Stuttgart New York

Penis Construction in Female-to-Male Transsexuals

D. R. Laub [1], W. Eicher [2], D. R. Laub II [1], and V. R. Hentz [1]

[1] Gender Dysphonia Program, Inc., 900 Welch Road, Suite 402, Palo Alto, CA 94304, USA
[2] Frauenklinik, Diakonissenkrankenhaus Mannheim, Speyerer Straße 91–93, 6800 Mannheim 1

What greater loss of body image is there than absence or loss of the penis? Greater losses exist, of course, but given the major deficit of loss of penis and the technical complexity involved in its restoration, one may state that the challenge for the reconstructive genitourinary surgeon in the 1980s is the formation of a penis with (a) sensitivity, (b) ability to urinate in a standing position, (c) passable to good appearance, and (d) ability for intromission in sexual intercourse. Gilbert has enunciated these criteria on several occasions, at meetings and on instructional courses.

The techniques for achieving the construction of a penis are evolving rapidly. The techniques for reconstruction, for gender dysphoria, and for traumatic amputation are similar in principle and can be discussed together.

The professionals who have worked in the field of gender dysphoria for a number of years have become familiar with this disease entity, and most workers have come to believe that the gender dysphoria patient carries a discrepancy that is as valid an indication for surgery as that in the intersex patient. The lack of wholeness, or failure of integration, of the gender dysphoria patient lies in the difference between the gender of the body and that of the mind.

The surgeon adjusts the anatomy of the body after legal, economic, social, sexual, and psychological adjustments are complete in the gender of choice, whereas the task of the social scientist is to determine the true gender and whether a particular patient is appropriate for surgery. Workers approach the patients with the attitude that the principles of rehabilitation should be used: that interdisciplinary talent is needed, that patients must enter society as workers, and that self-rehabilitation is superior to help given by others. The surgeons change the body to fit what has been determined to be the real, or true, or best gender. As Edgerton (1982) has remarked: "We deal with gender confirmation surgery, not sex change surgery."

With this philosophy, the Harry Benjamin International Gender Dysphoria Association (HBIGDA) was born as a professional association in 1978 in order that the disciplines would be able to interchange information and, most importantly, to set down professional guidelines which help define the appropriate patients for surgery. The HBIGDA guidelines for gender confirmation surgery (Laub 1985; Walker et al. 1985) have begun to be accepted by the legal profession, third-party insurance payers, and the medical professions, and also in the malpractice "arena." The guidelines contain criteria prerequisite for the diagnosis of gender dysphoria. Two social scientists, one with a PhD or equivalent, must participate in the diagnosis. One of them must have known the patient over a 6-

Plastic Surgery in the Sexually Handicapped
Eds.: W. Eicher/Kubli/Herms

month period. The patient must have had the feelings of being in the wrong body for at least 2 years. The criteria for surgery are (a) recommendation in writing by two behavioral scientists, one of whom has known the patient in a therapeutic relationship for 6 months; (b) a successful cross-living test over a 1-year period; and (c) legal, social, psychological, sexual, and (exogenous) endocrine success during the cross-living. Before any surgical gender reassignment is performed, appropriate monitoring of other medical conditions, as well as the effects of the hormones upon the liver and other organ systems, should be accomplished. The above should be appropriately documented.

Obviously, the rearrangement of the female body to the male is performed on those patients whose true, or most appropriate, gender has been determined to be male, and where the patient is already successful in life as a male.

Presented here is a menu of surgery options in the interests of a broad perspective. Naturally enough, the authors' choices are emphasized. Postmodern phalloplasty is preferred because it meets most of the criteria proposed by Gilbert. Postmodern phalloplasty (plan A) consists of the Chinese flap (Gao 1980, 1983; Song 1982, Yang et al. 1982) the standard midline abdominal flap, and a split-thickness skin graft. An alternative plan (plan B) is metaoidioplasty, which is available for gender dysphoria patients only: it utilizes the existing local tissue of the female external genitalia to fashion the male external genitalia. Another alternative (plan C) is the midline abdominal flap (without the radial forearm free flap). In this plan, devices are used to achieve sensory, intercourse, and urinary function (Figs. 9, 10).

Postmodern Phalloplasty

The donor tissues for postmodern phalloplasty are as follows (Fig. 1):

1. The Chinese flap (Chang et al. 1984; Gao 1980, 1983; Song 1982; Sun and Huang 1985; Yang et al. 1981) or radial forearm free flap (Heindl and Stock 1982)
2. A delayed transfer abdominal fasciocutaneous flap (6), partly based on the superficial external pudendal artery
3. A split-thickness skin graft

The Chinese (radial forearm) flap is exploited (Hentz 1985) for its:

1. Relatively hair-free skin to form the urethra
2. Superb blood supply – the huge radial artery (Song 1982; Yang et al. 1981) with fasciocutaneous perforators
3. The lateral antebrachial cutaneous nerve of the forearm, a continuation of the musculocutaneous nerve
4. Relatively "inexpensive," but nicely innervated, skin from the distal palmar aspect of the forearm to form the glans (Fig. 2).

The postmodern method utilizes the deep pudendal nerve for microsurgical fascicular neurorrhaphy to the lateral antebrachial cutaneous nerve. This hookup provides cerebral erotic connections. The lateral antebrachial cutaneous nerve terminates, with moderately acute nerve endings, in the "intelligent" glabrous skin at the base of the thumb. (This term, connoting a higher degree of sensibility

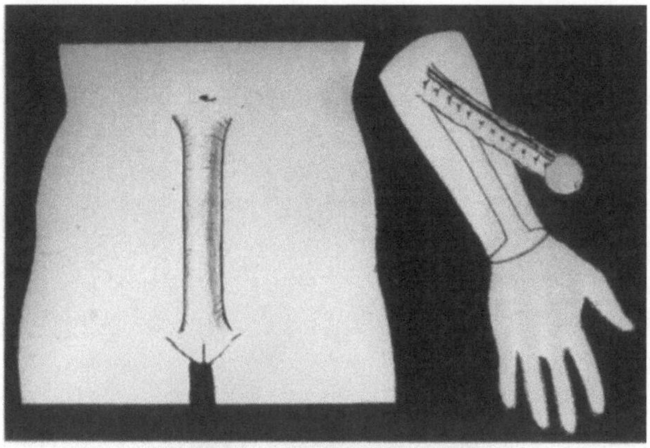

Fig. 1. The ingredients for postmodern phalloplasty

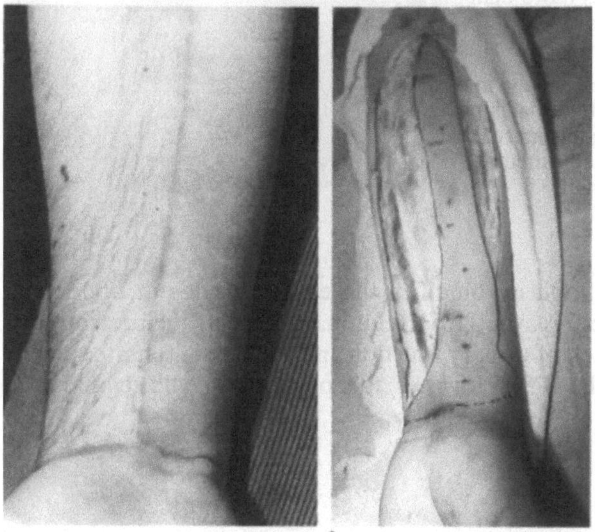

a b

Fig. 2a, b. A small Chinese or radial forearm flap, usually 25 × 3 cm, is combined with the standard abdominal tube. The donor sites for both are closed primarily without skin graft

and better information available to the cerebrum, was popularized by J.K. Terzis.) This patch of skin forms part of the glans penis (Zocchi et al. 1983).

Postmodern phalloplasty exploits the tubed abdominal flap (Laub 1980) for:

1. Good cosmetic appearance of the shaft. The thick split-thickness skin graft on the outside of the tube pedicle provides a glabrous, smooth, homogeneous, tight, "nonblobby" appearance.
2. A second, skin-lined tunnel for baculum placement for intercourse.
3. The Bulk required for normal cosmetic appearance, which is usually not available with the radial forearm flap alone.

This tube is raised as a midline bipedicle flap (Fig. 3) and formed into an inside-out tube (Fig. 4). A split-thickness skin graft is placed around it, on Scarpa's fascia, which is now on the external surface of the tube. This flap is employed by Davies (1972), Birdsell and Hentz (1973), and Laub (1980), but its anatomic basis has only recently been described by Patil et al. (1987).

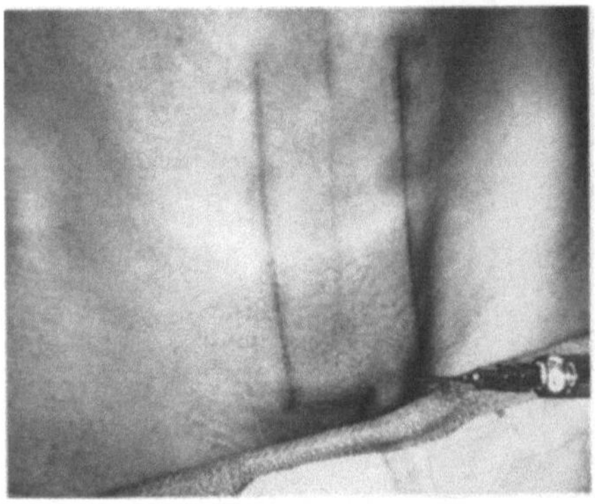

Fig. 3. Stage I incisions. The distance between incisions usually varies more than in this case. See text for details ("Technique")

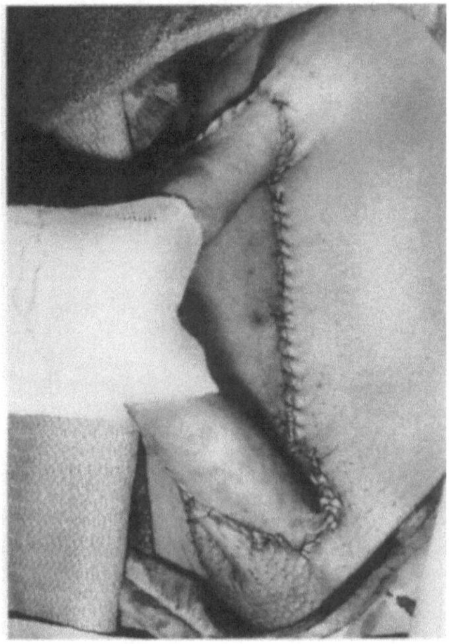

Fig. 4. The conclusion of stage I results in a bipedicle, inside out, covered with a skin graft, with abdominal forming an internal tunnel, which is hairy and usually used as needed for a stiffener or baculum

Thus, postmodern phalloplasty modifies the earlier inside-out abdominal phalloplasty, by adding the forearm flap, to eliminate some of the previous disadvantages, inlcuding (a) lack of urinary function and (b) lack of sensate skin for erotic function (Dubin et al. 1979). However, this phalloplasty still requires two stages.

Technique

In the first stage, the standard abdominal tube flap is formed as a longitudinal inside-out bipedicle flap (Fig. 4). This flap is partly random but relies on some axial pattern blood supply from the paired superficial external pudendal arteries and veins. Certain technical considerations are worth noting:

1. The tube is usually designed to be 15 cm long, with one pedicle base at the desired penile position (in transsexuals, usually the level of the cleft of the labia majora), and extending up to the infraumbilical area (Fig. 3).
2. The superficial external pudendal artery is located just beneath Scarpa's fascia, at the level of the symphysis pubis. In transsexual surgery, it would be found just superjacent to the round ligament (the homologue to the spermatic cord) 1.5 cm superior to the cleft of the labia majora. This vessel should be carefully preserved.
3. The superficial inferior epigastric arteries are severed, as they are located superior to the base of the pedicle.
4. The subcutaneous tissue varies in thickness in the area donated to the tube. It is thick at the suprapubic area, thin just superior to the mons, and of medium

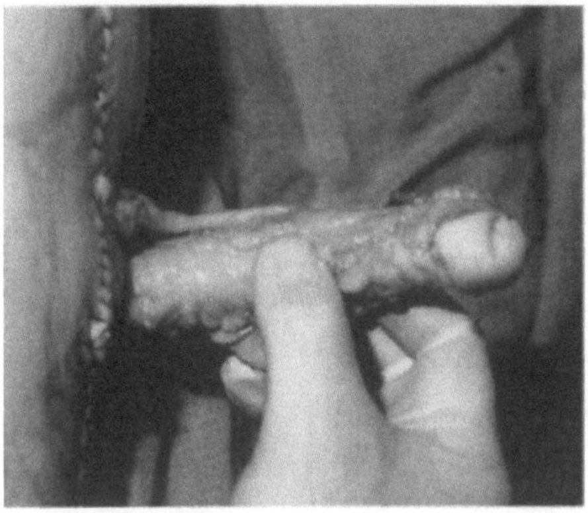

Fig. 5. The Chinese flap is formed into a penoid while still on the forearm

thickness at the infraumbilical area. Therefore, for the shaft to be of uniform diameter, the "parallel" lines of the paramedian incision must be drawn at varying distances apart. The incisions are further apart (8 cm) in thin tissue (pinch test + 3 cm) and closer together (5 cm) in tissue with pinch test greater than 3 cm.

5. The split-thickness skin graft may be thick: 0.018 in.
6. Scarpa's fascia is the deep layer of the superficial fascia and bears a longitudinal arcade of vessels. This vasculature makes this tissue a better recipient bed for skin grafts than the superficial fatty layer, Camper's fascia.

Between the first and second stages, 10–12 weeks are allowed. The second stage combines the radial forearm flap transfer with the release of the upper attachment of the bipedicle. The free flap is outlined on the glabrous skin of the palmar aspect of the forearm (Fig. 2). It is taken 2.5–3.5 cm wide and is formed into a tube while still on the forearm (Fig. 5). The fascia, which is taken 2 cm wider than the skin, is wrapped around the tube. No muscles are removed. The veins taken with the flap do not always include the cephalic vein, but rather those veins that are propitious, e.g., venae comitantes or superficial veins. The radial artery is usually anastomosed to the deep inferior epigastric artery, and the flap's veins to the venae comitantes of the deep inferior epigastric. In one case, anastomoses were made directly to the femoral artery and saphenous vein. The inguinal ligament may be (but usually is not) severed to prevent compromise of the blood supply. The lateral antebrachial nerve of the flap is attached to the deep pudendal nerve with microsurgical fascicular repair technique (Fig. 6). Debulking of the abdominal tube is needed to make room for the radial forearm flap, or some additional skin graft may be necessary to cover the inside-out forearm flap.

Abdominoplasty, and preparation for anastomosis to the urethra, may also be done in this stage but would increase the potential for complications because anticoagulant medication (aspirin) may be used for management of the microvascular anastomosis. Obviously, there are many permutations of the staging; a plan may be tailored to the patient's needs and the surgeon's experience. Certain considerations, however, ought to be kept in mind:

1. Urinary anastomosis is the most complication-prone aspect of the phalloplasty. In order to avoid infection and fistula formation, the neourethra is

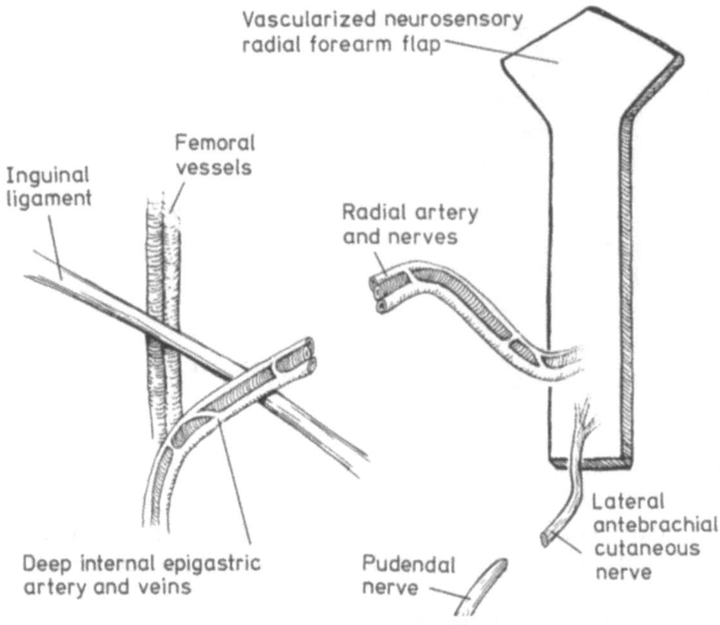

Fig. 6. The microhookups. The epigastric vessels may safely be allowed to remain subjacent to the inguinal ligament

not anastomosed to the urinary meatus in stage II, although this might easily be done at this time. The tissues are placed in proximity, leaving a fistula by intent. A silicone Jackson-Pratt 15-F drain is placed through the urethroplasty. This allows improved skin hygiene by irrigation with antiseptic or antibiotic solutions.

2. One month later, the urinary meatus and the neourethra can be anastomosed in a minor procedure. The principles developed in hypospadias correction are useful in designing flaps in this stage. In the transsexual patient, a flap is raised from the anterior vagina to extend from the female urinary meatus to the distal neourethra. This flap, as described by Bouman (1985), Thompson and Staffon (1960) and Thompson (1971), prevents a suture line in this area, which is vulnerable to fistulae because of urinary turbulence.
3. Closed (needle) suprapubic urethrostomy, although technically simpler than perineal urethrostomy, does not completely empty the bladder and may stimulate bladder spasm.
4. The split-thickness skin graft placed on the externalized Scarpa's fascia in the abdominal flap produces good cosmetic appearance (Fig. 7) but is completely denervated. Most innervated flaps have an excessively flaccid or "blobby" appearance.
5. The skin at the base of the thumb, which is used to form the glans penis, may be the least "expensive" donor site which provides specialized, sensitive nerve endings.

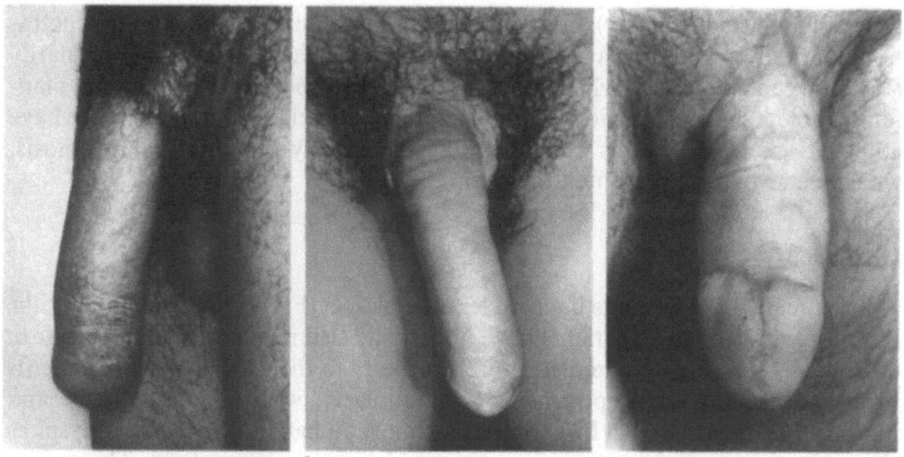

a b c

Fig. 7 a–c. Examples of the standard abdominal tube. The radial forearm flap may be added as a third stage to form the composite penis (postmodern phalloplasty)

Results

Six patients have undergone postmodern phalloplasty (Table 1). Two have experienced reinnervation of the glans. One patient especially has exquisite sensation in this area and has intercourse daily. One of these patients uses a baculum, but the others instead grasp the base of the penis, inhibiting venous drainage. The in-

Table 1. Experience with standard and postmodern phalloplasty

Surgery	No. of cases
Standard abdominal tube	180
Postmodern phalloplasty	6
Traumatic loss (tree shredder)	1
Female-to-male transsexual [a]	5

[a] Gender dysphoria syndrome.

Table 2. The incidence of morbidity in early cases of postmodern phalloplasty

Morbidity	No. of cases
Flap loss, total or partial	0
Venous occlusion ("take back")	1
Abscess, perineum	1
Fistula, urinary	2
Poor nerve regrowth [a]	2

[a] Not fully assessed.

flow of blood (radial artery) then makes the organ tumescent enough for penetration in a well-prepared partner. Forearm donor sites have been closed primarily (Fig. 2) except in one case where a skin graft was used because of an error in planning. Table 2 shows the incidence of infection and fistulae in early cases. We have adjusted our technique (as above) to allow for delay of urinary anastomosis, which seems to have prevented these complications.

Discussion

Approximately 195 patients have undergone plan C (Fig. 7), the abdominal tube flap. Almost 30 of these patients have undergone electrolysis of the pubic hair in an area large enough to complete a urethroplasty to the glans penis. Six patients have undergone plan A, postmodern phalloplasty, with abdominal tube and modified Chinese or radial forearm flap. Almost all patients had gender dysphoria syndrome except for a trauma patient and a micropenis patient. The gender dysphoria patients are by and large referred by the Gender Dysphoria Program of Palo Alto, Inc. [a California Foundation (501.C.3) organized in 1980 to assist patients with gender dysphoria syndrome, and to carry out public education in this area]. Selection criteria for surgery are more stringent than the minimal standards of the Harry Benjamin International Gender Dysphoria Association (Laub 1985; Walker et al. 1985). This professional association has set down guidelines accepted by the medical and legal professions, and the insurance industry.

The patient must be recommended for the surgery by two behavioral scientists, in writing. One of these must have known the patient in a professional psychotherapeutic relationship for 6 months. The patient must have been completely and successfully living in the genetically opposite sex role for at least 1 year – passing the "real-life" test. Prior to the surgical gender reassignment, the patient must have accomplished hormonal sex reassignment, which is of both diagnostic and therapeutic value. Hormonal treatment requires physical examination, and liver and blood chemistries measured yearly. In their recommendation, the two advocates must inform the surgeon not only that the 1 year of cross-living has been successful, but that the essential diagnostic features of the condition have been present continuously for 2 years or more: demonstration of discomfort in the gender role, the urge to rid the self of genitalia, freedom from psychosis, and the intense desire to change. The patients must realize that surgery is not the sole solution to their psychosocial adaptation, or even the solution to body-image deficits.

The high cost and complication of surgical therapy for gender dysphoria syndrome are valid negative considerations. But these must be placed in perspective with other high-tech major rehabilitative surgical projects such as hip replacement, kidney transplant, spinal surgery, or coronary artery bypass grafts. Gender dysphoria surgery compares well with these projects, especially in their developmental stages. In well-selected cases, gender dysphoria is truly rehabilitative: an individual is transformed from a state of relative disability to that of a productive, better adjusted member of society (Edgerton 1984).

With our knowledge of the embryology of the external genitalia, and with plastic surgery's newly acquired ability to transfer distant tissue in one stage via microvascular anastomoses, it may only be a matter of time and effort before our dreams regarding construction of the phallus are realized.

We have capitalized on work by Gilbert and Horton indicating the role of the deep pudendal nerve in the circuit of erotogenic sensation. Transferring the clitoral nerve to the surgically created glans penis uses the existing functional connections of the deep pudendal nerve to the sensorium. Terzis and others have demonstrated that the two-point discrimination of skin grafts is better in glabrous than in hairy skin (Dykes et al. 1984; Zocchi et al. 1983; J.K. Terzis, personal communication). Although a free flap is not strictly analogous to an experimental skin graft, glabrous skin for the glans is clearly preferable, and an effort is made to utilize relatively hair-free skin for surfacing the shaft of the penis.

In developing this phalloplasty technique, we have assumed without any firm research basis (other than the knowledge that the most sensitive area of the penis is the corona; Gilbert et al. 1986) that the sensation in the glans is more important than that in the shaft of the penis.

Prior to use of the forearm flap, experience was gained in a series of 150 phalloplasties (Laub 1986). These phalloplasties were surgically straightforward, with very few complications in the latter part of the series, and many were cosmetically acceptable (Fig. 7). They did not, however, provide a functional male urethra. This present series, while consisting of few patients, is well grounded in our previous work and should present few complications.

This phalloplasty is our attempt to satisfy the criteria proposed by Gilbert, but it is still imperfect (Fig. 8). It has the potential to achieve these goals with the improvements evolving through experience. Postmodern phalloplasty now achieves (a) erotic sensibility, (b) neourethra, (c) moderately good appearance, and (d) ability for intromission.

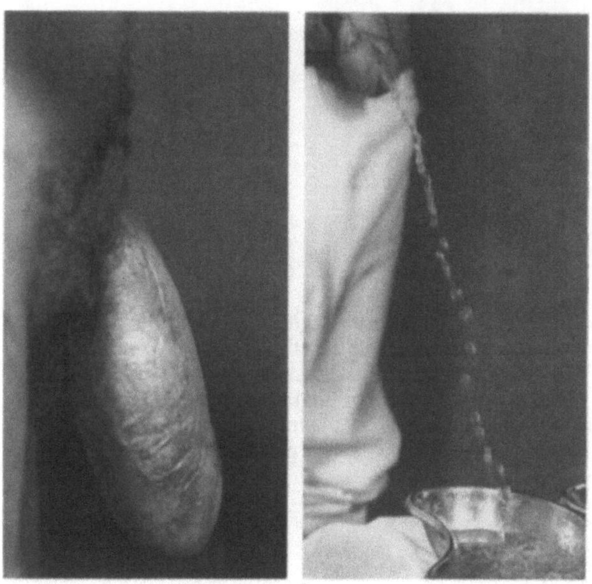

a b

Fig. 8 a, b. Results of postmodern phalloplasty (plan A) performed for total amputation in tree-shredding machine

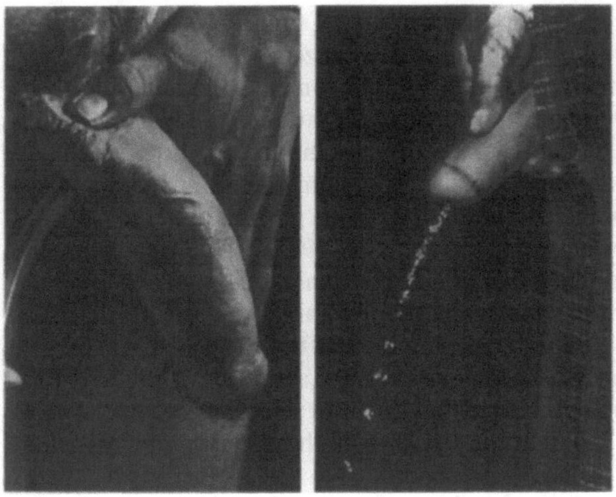

a b

Fig. 9 a, b. The urinary assist device (UAD; Precision Ocular Prosthetics, Redwood City, California) consists of silicone tubing of relatively large caliber, which conducts the urine tunnel of the pedicle. The patient stands to urinate and uses the male public urinals. He wears the UAD in his underclothing and holds the reservoir directly under the (female) urinary meatus at the time of micturition. Use of this device requires custom fitting and a certain amount of practice to achieve the required psychomotor coordination

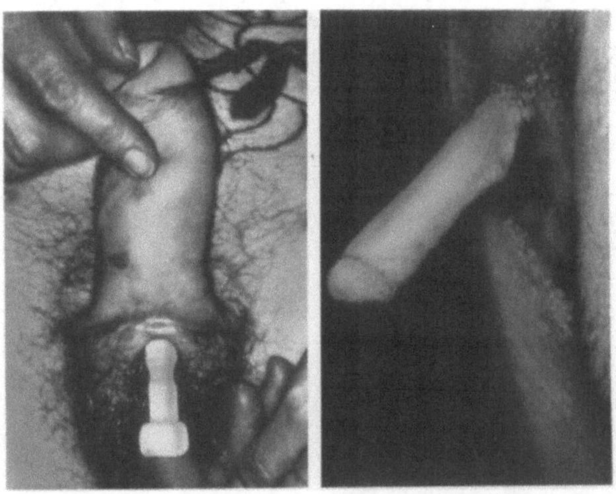

a b

Fig. 10 a, b. The baculum (OS penis; Precision Ocular Prosthetics, Redwood City, California) is inserted at time of sexual intercourse to achieve a stiffening for intromission, and to achieve sexual stimulation. The patient is required to direct the penis by grasping at the base of the penis. The proximal portion of the device stimulates the more erotogenic structures at the clitoris and labia minora. Custom tailoring is helpful to prevent telescoping of the device out the meatus at the glans, an event which is potentially dangerous to the partner

As mentioned above, the alternative most frequently chosen by patients in previous years has been the two-stage abdominal tube pedicle flap alone, without the free flap, which we term plan C. Function has been achieved by use of (a) the urinary assist device (Fig. 9) and (b) the baculum (Fig. 10).

Approximately 30 of 164 patients have undergone urethroplasty, with depilated local skin being used. This technique has been successful, but the 1-year period necessary for the electrolysis of this very sensitive tissue is a significant drawback. The skin which is to be used for the pedicle (9 × 15 cm on lower abdominal midline) and the 5-cm strip of skin of the pubis and upper labia majora are depilated at least 12 weeks prior to surgery. The urethroplasty uses principles and techniques similar to those for hypospadias closure.

Metaoidioplasty

Metaoidioplasty (plan B) is defined as the surgical change toward male external genitalia, the term being derived from the Greek. In embryonic development, the external genitalia of both male and female come from the same precursor, as is shown in Figs. 11, 12. For purposes of discussion, consider that female external anatomy would become male external anatomy if appropriate hormones were present in utero. These chemicals are not available for use by our endocrinology colleagues for our adult patients. Testosterone will only enlarge the clitoris of the adult female body to a certain size.

In this technique (Fig. 13), the clitoris is moved 3 cm anteriorly to the penis position. The labia majora are moved 3 cm posteriorly and fused together into the scrotum configuration. The external aspects of the labia minora are converted into ventral penis skin, and the internal aspects into urethral mucosa.

Female derivative		Primordial structure		Male derivative
Clitoris Corpora cavernosa Glans clitoridis	←	Genital tubercle	→	Penis Corpora cavernosa Glans penis
Internal aspects of labia minora	←	Urethral fold	→	Corpus spongiosum (enclosing penile urethra)
Labia majora and external aspects of labia minora	←	Labioscrotal swellings	→	Scrotum and ventral epidermis of penis
Paraurethral glands (of Skene)	←	Urogenital sinus	→	Prostate
Bartholin's gland				Bulbourethral glands (of Cowper)
Vagina (lower)				Prostatic utricle (vagina masculina)

Fig. 11. Male and female homologues in the external genitalia

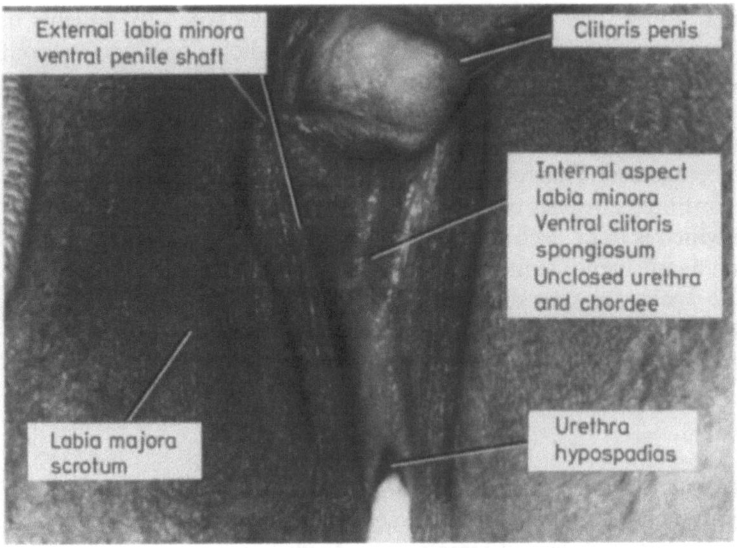

Fig. 12. The external anatomy of the male and female are derived from the same tissue. The male structures are the female structures which have been transformed by the influence of intrauterine hormones. Hormones given to adult women do not complete the metamorphosis to male external genitalia. Surgery attempts to mimic the natural process

The chordee is released and excised according to the principles of hypospadias surgery.

Testicular prostheses are inserted into the neoscrotum. The mons pubis and/or the lower abdominal subcutaneous and skin excess are removed by a small abdominoplasty, i.e., by excision, suction-assisted lipectomy, and rotation of this tissue to the deficits caused by the movement of the labia majora. This mini lower abdominoplasty reduces the feminine mons veneris and also allows the patient to visualize the little penis better, without the obstruction of the mons veneris or a small abdominal pannus. The Laub urethroplasty reaches only the length of the penis and does not form the portion of the urethra connecting the phallus with the existing female external urinary meatus. The "membranous" urethra from the base of the penis through the scrotum must be reconstituted with full-thickness skin graft at a second stage. The Bouman-Thompson flap (Bouman 1985; Thompson and Staffon 1960; Thompson 1971) almost provides enough tissue from anterior vagina to make this connection.

Fig. 13 a–h. Metaoidioplasty. **a** Female external genitalia after 2 years of exogenous hormone administration, which enlarges the clitoris to a certain size only. **b** The inner surface of labia minora, which can easily convert to male urethra. **c** The incisions. The labia majora, pedicled by posterior blood supply from the internal pudendal system, are moved 2–2.5 cm posteriorly. **d** The clitoris is moved 2 cm anteriorly, and the tissue deficit on its ventral surface is surfaced with the labia minora. **e** A diagram of the above. **f–h** Postsurgery results

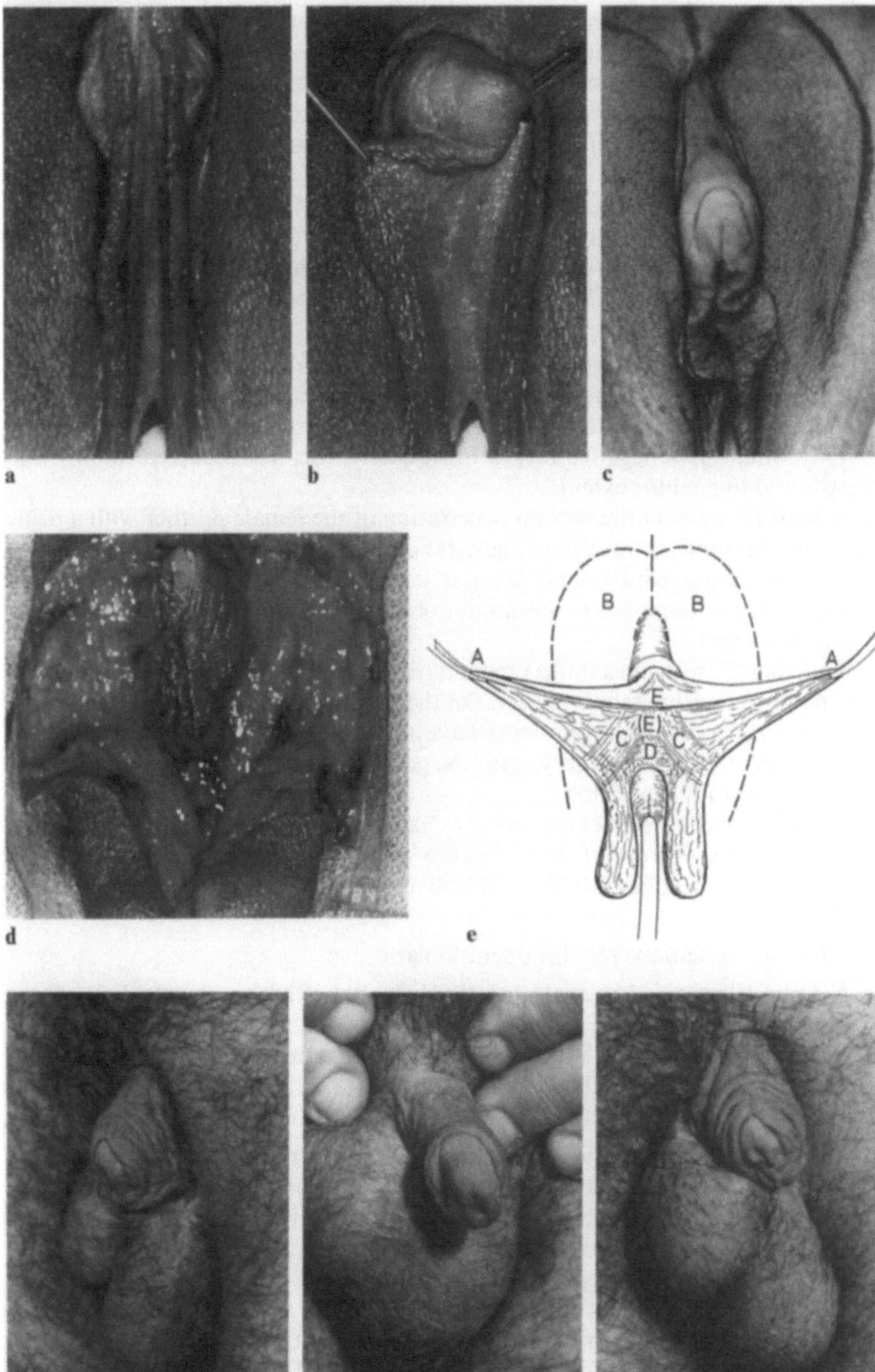
a
b
c
B
B
A
A
E
(E)
C
C
D
d
e
f
g
h

In the Eicher clitorispenoid operation, the deficiency in the Laub procedures is remedied by extending the urinary passage to the tip of the clitoris after refreshing and partial resection of the small labia. The internal aspects of the labia minora are converted into urethral epithelium, being closed over a catheter forming a urethral tube. (*Clitorispenoid* refers to the clitoris being transformed into a penislike structure.)

In reviewing 65 operated cases, it has become clear that when the patients were offered the choice between the various phalloplasty techniques, certain patient objectives were more predominant in the population that elected metaoidioplasty or clitorispenoid surgery. Clitorispenoid/metaoidioplasty is usually indicated for or elected by:

1. Individuals who have been married to a woman in the nonoperative condition for 2–15 years. These female-to-males have been practicing a sexual union which involves the clitoris of the male partner. In this situation, loss of sensitivity would be a negative result. Fortunately, this has occurred in only one case, and to a minor extent.
2. Persons for whom intravaginal penetration of the female partner with a penis is unimportant. Intravaginal penetration with the penis that is surgically formed using a clitoris and labia is possible but is generally not reliably achieved, and therefore it should not be predicted, anticipated, or warranted preoperatively.
   Note that those using a dildo preoperatively may continue to use the dildo for penetration postmetaoidioplasty. On the other side of the coin, those using a dildo preoperatively may desire to have a large penis made by local abdominal tube flap or by microsurgery, with the goal in mind to achieve a more natural replacement for the dildo.
3. Cases where the "least expensive sex change" is the overriding consideration. In such cases, this one-stage procedure (which does not involve microsurgery transplantation) does fulfill the objectives of a legal sex change with minimal surgical costs.

Negative indications for this operation are:

1. A desire to obtain the usual archetypal symbol of maleness, which is a large penis.
2. A desire for the ability to have intravaginal intercourse.
3. Necessity to urinate in the standing position. (This may be fulfilled in certain cases, e.g., clitorispenoid.)

At the Eighth International Congress of the Harry Benjamin International Gender Dysphoria Association meeting in Minneapolis, USA, Bouman (1985), of the Department of Plastic Surgery at the Free University in Amsterdam, reported a method of extending the urinary meatus out to the position of a penoscrotal hypospadias (as preparation for phalloplasty). His tecniques are in some ways similar to those of Eicher.

The operation has been performed in the past not only by Eicher and Laub but also by R. DeMuth and E. Tank (Departments of Plastic Surgery and Urology at the University of Oregon), and by an Italian surgeon mentioned at the Society for the Scientific Study of Sex meeting in Washington, DC in 1982.

Clitorispenoid/metaoidioplasty addresses the tissue deficits from the point of view of using the same tissue that is used in embryologic development. The operation satisfies the legal requirements for sex confirmation surgery, while producing a penis which is acutely sensitive. It has the appearance of a small boy's penis, or the penis that may be seen in locker rooms after a very cold shower (Fig. 13).

Conclusion

Many methods now exist for construction of the penis. We have presented three of these – metaoidioplasty or clitorispenoid, postmodern phalloplasty, and standard abdominal tube – with an effort to compare advantages and disadvantages in order to allow the patient and surgeon to tailor their choices accordingly. We are sure that improvements will be forthcoming, as many disciplines are contributing to the breakthroughs.

References

Birdsell D, Hentz VR (1973) Phalloplasty. In: Proceedings of the Harry Benjamin International Gender Dysphoria Association Conference, Stanford University

Bouman J (1985) Phalloplasty using existing tissue. Paper presented at the Harry Benjamin International Gender Dysphoria Association meeting, Minneapolis, Minn., September 1985

Chang Ti-Sheng, Hwang Wen-Yi (1984) Forearm flap in one-stage reconstruction of the penis. Plast Reconstr Surg 74(2):251–258

Davies D (1972) Reconstruction of the penis. Paper presented at the American Association of Plastic Surgeons meeting, San Francisco, CA

Dubin BT, Sato RI, Laub DR (1979) Results of phalloplasty. Plast Reconstr Surg 64:163

Dykes RW, Terzis JK, Turnbull BG (1984) Properties of mechanoreceptive fibres serving skin grafts transferred to the hands of adult baboon (*Papio anubis*). J Physiol (Lond) 357:1–22

Edgerton M (1982) Presidential address. Given at Harry Benjamin International Gender Dysphoria Association meeting. Bordeaux

Edgerton ME (1984) The role of surgery in the treatment of transsexualism. Ann Plast Surg 13(6):473

Eicher W (1984) Transsexualismus, Möglichkeiten und Grenzen der Geschlechtsumwandlung (Transsexualism, Possibilities and Limits of Sexual Transformation). Fischer, Stuttgart New York

Gao XS (1980) Reconstruction of the penis: report of four cases (in Chinese). Chung-Hua Wai Ko Tsa Chih 18:67–68

Gao XS (1984) One-stage Reconstruction of the penis with free skin flap from the forearm (in Chinese). Chung Hua I Hsuch Tsa Chih 64:470–473

Gilbert D, Horton C, Terzis J, Devine C, Williams M, Grossman J (1986) Phallic re-innervation via the internal pudendal nerve. In: Mathes SJ (ed) Plastic surgery forum, vol 9. Am Soc Plast Reconstr Surg, Inc, Chicago, pp 39–40

Heindl E, Stock W (1982) The forearm flap. Plast Reconstr Surg 70:336–442

Hentz VR (1985) The versatile forearm flap. Paper presented at the American Association of Plastic Surgery meeting, San Diego, CA, May 1985

Laub DR (1980) Random pedicle flap for phalloplasty. Paper presented at plastic surgery education foundation symposium, University of East Virginia

Laub DR (1985) Letter to the editor. Ann Plast Surg
Laub DR (1986) Phalloplasty with forearm flap. Paper presented at Texas Plastic Surgery Society Annual Meeting, Dallas, TX, May 1986
Patil UA, Dias AD, Thatte RL (1987) The anatomic basis of the SEPA flap. Br J Plast Surg 40:342–347
Song RY (1982) Total reconstruction of the male genitalia. Chinese Plast Surg 9:97
Sun G, Huang J (1985) One-stage reconstruction of the penis with composite iliac crest and lateral groin flap. Ann Plast Surg 15:519–528
Tank ES, DeMuth RJ, Rosenberg S (1982) Reconstruction following amputation of the penis in children. J Urol 128:386–388
Thompson IM (1971) Results of vaginal flap urethroplasty in hermaphrodites. J Urol 105:456–459
Thompson IM, Staffon R (1960) An operative technique for the management of certain defects of pseudohermaphroditism. J Urol 84:406–408
Walker PA, Berger JC, Green R, Laub DR, Reynolds CL Jr, Wollman L (Founding Committee of the Harry Benjamin Gender Dysphoria Association) (1985) Standards of care: the hormonal and surgical sex reassignment of gender dysphoria persons. Arch Sex Behav 14:75–90
Yang G, Chen B, Gao Y (1981) The forearm free skin flap transplantation. Chung-Hua I Hsueh Tsa Chih 61:139
Zocchi M, Teich-Alasia S, Stella M (1983) Etude functionelle et morphologique de la résensibilisation de lambeaux cutanés transplantés. Rev Stomatol Chir Maxillofac 84:85–92

Results and Follow-up of Surgically Transformed Transsexuals

V. Herms

Abteilung Gynäkologie und Geburtshilfe, Kreiskrankenhaus,
8765 Erlenbach/Main, FRG

The therapeutic approach to be adopted for patients with a transsexual syndrome continues to be a subject of debate in the light of the present state of research. Psychotherapy with the objective of freeing transsexual patients from their wish to change their sex has hitherto largely proven to be unsuccessful. The commonest method of treatment currently is to administer hormones for a certain period prior to surgical sexual reassignment. In the Federal Republic of Germany, the sex change operation has been a precondition for a person to be able to change his or her legal sexual status since the law relating to transsexuals came into force in 1980. All in all, there is little consensus with regard to the positive or negative effects of the sexual reassignment operation as far as the psychological and social stability of the individual is concerned. In the first phase, the majority of investigations gave somatic indications that the reassignment operation had a positive effect. Most of the patients examined were assessed to be psychologically and socially stable. Later investigations showed the limitations with regard to the therapeutic success of the operation.

An intense controversy over the extent to which the sex reassignment operation actually does have positive effects on the psychological and social integration of transsexual patients was sparked off by the work of Meyer and Reter in 1979. These authors came to the conclusion that the psychological and social stability of surgically treated transsexuals does not differ substantially from that of transsexuals who have not undergone the operation. On the other hand, more recent catamneses all tend to indicate a relatively good social and psychological integration of transsexuals who have undergone surgery.

Springer, an Austrian psychiatrist (1981), is fundamentally against the indication for a sex transformation having the character of an "emergency therapy." He regards associated threats by patients to mutilate themselves or to commit suicide as usually an attempt to coerce doctors, and he researched the cases of genital self-mutilation well described in the international literature, which, in many instances, were not the result of transsexual wishes, but came about in the course of an acute or chronic psychotic process.

There is a further reason for Springer's doubts regarding the necessity for sexual reassignment operations: Springer criticizes the fact that, as he sees it, a circular line of reasoning has caused a myth to develop, namely, that patients with a transsexual syndrome are psychotherapeutically untreatable. He demonstrates that it is always the same authors who are quoting each other, sometimes without indicating whether they have tried any psychotherapeutic approaches themselves at all, or simply neglecting contrary opinions and reports of successful psycho-

Plastic Surgery in the Sexually Handicapped
Eds.: W. Eicher/Kubli/Herms

therapy for the desire to change sex. According to Benedetti (1981), however, the split identity of the transsexual is persistent: it cannot be altered by any psychotherapy.

In our catamnestic investigation, we were able to reexamine 45 male-to-female and 19 female-to-male transsexuals from a total of 85 transsexuals who had undergone reassignment surgery between 1975 and 1982 in the University in Heidelberg. The basic reaction to the invitation to participate in the catamnestic investigation was rather negative. Initially, one-third of the patients did not respond to the written invitation at all. Many patients of both sexes wished, following their genital transformation operation, not to be reconfronted with their case history if at all possible.

Several years' prior "practice" living in the role of a member of the opposite sex proved to be a good selection criterion in deciding whether an operation was the suitable method of treatment. The male-to-female transsexuals had on average a considerably longer period of practice than the originally female patients. Accordingly, some of them were very natural in their gestures and in the way they dressed, made themselves up, spoke, and moved about. The appearance and demeanor of these patients facilitated their adaptation. On the other hand, the female-to-male transsexuals adapted themselves on average more quickly because, in a manner typical of their adopted sex, they attached less importance to their external appearance than the male-to-female transsexuals. The following factors constituted negative selection criteria in our group in considering the necessity for genital corrective surgery: (a) personality disorders of a paranoid or querulous nature; (b) totally unsuitability – in terms of appearance, demeanor, and physiognomy – for adaptation to the outward appearance of the opposite sex; (c) loss of a sense of reality, e.g., in the case of decompensating borderline structure; or (d) advanced age of a patient (over 45 years).

About two-thirds of the patients of both sexes reexamined by us felt subjectively better than before the operation. In their case, a good-to-satisfactory harmonization between feelings of psychosexual affinity and physical appearance had taken place. In social terms, the effects of the operation tended to be less favorable for both sexes. Job difficulties or disappointed expectations with regard to a partnership were, however, seen by the transsexuals as of secondary importance and as something to be put up with.

After allowing for the few cases which in terms of the overall impression could be categorized as neither significantly improved nor worsened, a clear worsening of the patient's psychological condition, including social disadvantages, occurred in only a tiny minority of cases. Male-to-female transsexuals declined to have the genital transformation operation less often than female-to-male transsexuals.

At the time of their initial consultation with a physician, male-to-female transsexuals were on average 2 years older than the originally female patients. At the time of the operation, the male-to-female transsexuals were, on average, 6 years older than the originally female patients. It thus took the male-to-female transsexuals significantly longer to achieve their goal and undergo the operation. About half of the male-to-female transsexuals had to put up with a deterioration in their job situation, whereas this was not so in the case of the originally female patients.

The intensity of the patient's wish to undergo sexual transformation is in most cases assuaged by corrective genital surgery. Generally, most transsexuals feel much calmer, more stable, and more content after the operation. The inner strife – caused by the discrepancy between feelings of psychosexual affinity and physical sexual characteristics – that is responsible for the patient's suffering is significantly and positively influenced, being replaced by greater inner harmony. This subjective improvement in the patient's condition is, however, also substantially promoted by the recommended continued treatment with hormones of the opposite sex after the operation.

It is noticeable that many transsexuals, especially patients with paranoid and querulous personality traits, make an "error of nature" responsible for their dilemma in order to achieve their goal of an operation. If, according to these patients' subjective impressions, the preparatory examinations for the operation take too long, or if there are complications after the operation, or expectations of acceptance and recognition are disappointed, these patients vehemently attack society and the legal and medical institutions, blaming them for an unsuccessful adaptation to the new sexual role. In extreme cases, a pension is demanded as a kind of compensation because the patients have become "invalids" as a result of the operation. A tendency toward the politicization of transsexuals and the harboring of expectations of society becomes particularly evident in some transsexuals' reluctance to pay their bills. However, this is possibly an expression of the inability of many transsexuals to integrate their own masculine and feminine elements to form an individual unity. While at first, nature is made responsible for this inability, the cause is later often projected onto society. With many of the patients reexamined by our group, the operation can be regarded as palliative surgery, by means of which the discrepancy between feelings of psychosexual affinity and biological status – the symptom which is the source of the most suffering – is substantially reduced (Table 1).

The 58 male-to-female and 45 female-to-male transsexuals operated on by Eicher (1984) were reexamined between 3 months and 8 years after the operation. Data on 90% of the patients from both groups have been recorded. None of the patients regret having had the operation, and all of them would wish to undergo surgical sexual reassignment once more if faced with the same situation again. Generally, it can be said that the patients with the best surgical results express the greatest satisfaction and are also best adapted in terms of job and environment.

Table 1. Follow-up studies

	Individuals Interviewed	Percentage of transsexuals who did *not* regret operation
1. Eicher (1984)	103	100%
2. Fahrner, Kockott, Duran (1987)	32	100%
3. Hastings, Markland (1978)	25	100%
4. Herms (1987)	54	100%
5. Turner, Edlich, Edgerton (1978)	47	100%

In the case of the 10% of male-to-female transsexuals who suffered a vaginal stenosis or shortening of the vaginal passage, there was dissatisfaction with the local results, which naturally also impaired the capacity to experience satisfactory sexual relations. Of the male-to-female transsexuals with a functional vagina, 80% have the capacity to experience orgasm during intravaginal sexual intercourse. In the case of the female-to-male transsexuals, Eicher reports general satisfaction with the surgery performed. Each patient would again wish to undergo surgical sexual reassignment. All patients were clearly told prior to surgery that it is not possible to achieve a fully functional penis, and that an abdominal tubular pedicle flap penoid is not to be recommended. The patients who did not undergo phalloplastic surgery tend to be more stable and well-balanced in psychological terms. Most patients were able, after the transformation and the change in their legal sexual status, to live under reasonable socioeconomic conditions.

The 10 patients of Eicher's who have a clitoris penoid are all psychologically stabilized and do not regret this solution, which enables them to urinate while standing. However, the majority of them are waiting for the day when they might yet receive a normal-sized erectile penis. Eicher has not observed any cases of postoperative attempted suicide, schizophrenia, or severe depression. Turner et al. (1978) operated on 53 male-to-female transsexuals and followed up 47 cases for at least 1 year. All patients retained a positive attitude to their decision after the operation, were freed from anxieties after the operation, and felt more self-confident and socially adapted. None regretted the operation. Psychoses and suicides were not observed, although in about 50% of the cases surgical corrections were necessary.

Hastings and Markland (1978) examined 25 male-to-female transsexuals after 5 years. They came to the conclusion that the general level of success in terms of personal satisfaction, if not excellent, was good, and that therefore there was at that time no other means of treating transsexualism than by surgery.

In 1979, the above-mentioned catamnestic study carried out by Meyer and Reter (1978) at the Johns Hopkins University in Baltimore led to a suspension of surgical operations, and this caused worldwide confusion. In their study, Meyer and Reter compared transsexuals who had undergone surgical sexual reassignment with those who had not been operated on. They expressed their surprise that, while none regretted having had the operation, the patients who had undergone surgery were not actually in a better position than those who had not, in terms either of socioeconomic status or of their stability. They concluded that transsexuals do not benefit from the operation with regard to their social rehabilitation, although all those who had been properly advised and had undergone the operation were satisfied with the results. As it cannot be ruled out that a significant number of those who did not receive surgical therapy and could not be followed up further underwent surgery elsewhere, this study cannot clarify the question of whether surgical treatment of transsexuality is justified.

In one of the most recent catamnestic investigations (Kockott et al. 1987), 59 patients who had been diagnosed as transsexuals were examined; 32 of them had undergone surgical sexual reassignment. By and large, it was shown that the transsexuals who had undergone surgery live a well-adjusted life in social terms and are psychologically almost inconspicuous. This social and psychological stability improved between the time of diagnosis and the time of the catamnesis. It is interesting that in some cases improvements occur even before the sexual reassignment operation. In a comparison with the transsexuals who had not undergone surgery in the random sample, those who had had the operation manifested significantly fewer psychological and social problems.

It can today be regarded as certain that the sexual reassignment operation makes a substantial contribution toward psychosocial stability. This is, however, only true provided that there has been a thorough and accurate diagnosis and good consultation over an adequate period in preparation for the operation and the desired gender status.

The diagnostic phase serves to differentiate the transsexual syndrome from other disturbances with similar manifestations. Furthermore, the patient must be made aware of the consequences of the sexual reassignment operation. The therapeutic tasks during the real-life test involve the learning of adequate behavior patterns in the desired gender status. It is important to work on the problems associated with the social environment which arise as a result of the change of sex. In this connection, concrete plans of action, e.g., to achieve a change in the person's employment situation and the use of relaxation exercises, can be helpful. If difficulties exist with the family or other persons with whom the patient has a close relationship, these should be dealt with within the framework of the therapy. The therapeutic measures begun during the real-life test should also be continued after the operation. The subjects of partnership and sexuality would appear to be especially important in this context.

References

1. Benedetti G (1981) Transsexualismus in der Sicht der Psychoanalyse. Prax Psychother Psychosom 26:183–186
2. Eicher W (1984) Transsexualismus. Fischer, Stuttgart New York
3. Hastings D, Markland C (1978) Post-surgical adjustment of twenty-five transsexuals (male-to-female) in the University of Minnesota study. Arch Sex Behavior 7:327–335
4. Fahrner EM, Kockott G, Duran G (1987) Die psychosoziale Integration operierter Transsexueller. Der Nervenarzt 58:340–348
5. Meyer JK, Reter DJ (1979) Sex reassignment. Follow up. Arch Gen Psychiatr 36:1010–1015
6. Springer A (1981) Pathologie der geschlechtlichen Identität. Springer, Wien New York
7. Turner VG, Edlich RF, Edgerton M (1978) Male transsexualism. A review of genital surgical reconstruction. Amer J Obstet Gynec 132:119–133

Part 6: Penis Prosthesis in Impotence

Inflatable Penile Prostheses

F. Schreiter and J. Denil

Urological Department, Verbandskrankenhaus Martfeld, Dr. Moellerstraße 15,
5830 Schwelm, FRG

The use of penile prostheses is the oldest and best-known treatment of erectile dysfunction. In the last few years, alternative methods have been presented, i.e., self-injection of the corpora cavernosa with vasoactive drugs, ligature of the penile deep dorsal vein, and bypass operations to improve the arterial blood supply to the penis. Although increasingly popular, these alternative methods have not been able to reduce the number of prosthesis implantations in the long run. After a short initial drop, the implantation rate is again increasing worldwide. This is due to critical reports on the alternative treatments.

Ligation of the deep dorsal vein has become more and more controversial since it became known that venous leaks are situated not only in these veins but also in the corporal wall, the central vein, or glandulocavernosal shunts. In spite of some isolated good results, a critical review of the literature shows a long-term success rate of less than 50%.

Self-Injection of the corpora cavernosa, currently very popular, is not without risks. In about 10% of all patients, priapismlike prolonged erections have occurred, leading to irreparable damage to the corpora if not treated in time. Therefore, these patients have to be followed closely by physicians familiar with priapism management. A death caused by sepsis after inappropriate self-injection has recently been reported.

The revascularization procedures are limited to men aged under 50 years suffering from nongeneralized arterial disease. The vascular lesions must be localized by arteriography and bypassed in a time-consuming, delicate microsurgical operation, which has a success rate of 40%–60%. If it is successful, the patients natural erection, controlled by the normal physiological mechanism, will be restored. All the other treatments have the disadvantage of being more or less artificial or of not bringing back the naturally occurring erection. This is even more crucial in prosthetic surgery, and the surgeon has to mention it, thus avoiding false expectations on the part of the patient (Porst 1987; Wespes 1987).

The choice of the appropriate treatment of erectile dysfunction seems, then, to be a bigger problem for the urologist than ever before. The main question is how the chosen therapy benefits the patient. In spite of the newer methods, implantation of penile prostheses of various types will remain the most important treatment in the near future. The rodlike devices, which are relatively easy to implant, have become very popular all over the world. The inflatable devices offer a more "natural" erection and deflation, but because of their elevated price, the possible mechanical failures, and the more complicated operative procedure, they are confined to a few centers familiar with their management. Patient selection

Plastic Surgery in the Sexually Handicapped
Eds.: W. Eicher/Kubli/Herms

is of the utmost importance in their use, and this critical review of the history of inflatable prostheses and our experience with them will try to facilitate this selection.

History and Critical Review of Penile Implants

The first, totally rigid prosthesis, which was placed outside the corpora cavernosa, is now no longer used. Today, available intracorporal penile implants can be divided into semirigid or rodlike devices and those with a hydraulic mechanism. The latter can either use a separate reservoir and a pump connected to inflatable cylinders by tubes – the fully inflatable prostheses – or contain both control pump and reservoir in the cylinder itself – the so-called self-contained devices (Fig. 1).

Their apparently easy implantation and rather low price of the semirigid devices made them very popular all over the world. The most-used types are the Jonas silicone-silver prosthesis and the AMS 600 malleable prosthesis, which were conceived in the 1970s. Both are made of silicone rubber, with a wire inside that neutralizes the rebound forces of the rubber, allowing a steady state in each position. The erection is permanent, but the penis can be bent down- or sideward to conceal it under the clothes. These devices only differ in the kind of wire used. The AMS uses a solid stainless steel wire, and the jonas a twisted silver one, but both behave in the same way while being bent. In time, they tend to break the bending point, which is explained by the microstructure of the metal wire: if overstretched the atomic grid will not return to its former configuration (fixed deformation); if forced, the microstructure falls apart and the wire breaks. Every one of us has experienced this phenomenon when trying to break a steel wire by

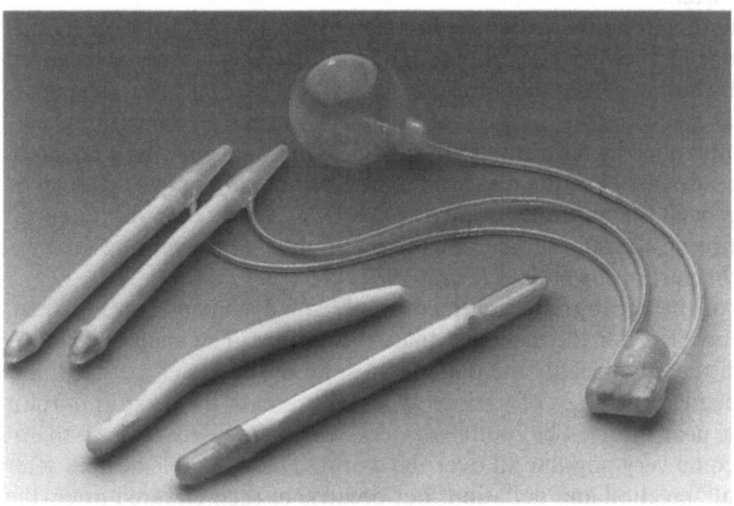

Fig. 1. The three different types of prosthesis: fully inflatable (*left*, IPP 700), semirigid (*middle*), and self-containing (*right*)

bending it up- and downward (Jonas 1983; Jonas and Jacobi 1980; Montague 1984; N. Kaula, personal communication, 1986).

The problem of breaking does not occur in the (also very popular) Small-Carrion prosthesis, developed in 1975, which is made of silicone rubber only. However, because of the permanent, inconcealable erection it produces, it must be considered obsolete. The Finney prosthesis or Surgitek-Flexirod device (1977) is a similarly constructed device, which, thanks to a weaker infrapubic part, can hang down. The main point of criticism here is the insufficient stability during intercourse. All semirigid devices have two common disadvantages: they exert a steady pressure on the corporal wall, which can lead to perforation, and they interfere with later endoscopic examination or surgery (Finney 1977, 1984; Small 1984).

Dissatisfaction with the semirigid implants led to the development of the hydraulic devices. The first of these was conceived in 1973 by Scott, Bradley, and Timm, and was the precursor of the AMS hydraulic prosthesis. In order to overcome the problems and failures observed, the device was constantly improved. In the course of this evolution, five different generations can be discerned (Kothari et al. 1972; Malloy et al. 1980; Schreiter 1974, 1985; Scott et al. 1973, 1983).

The first device involved the discomfort of utilizing two pumps and nonexpansive cylinders. It often showed leaks, valve failures, and a tendency toward deflating during intercourse. It was rather an experimental device and was implanted in only a few patients in 1973. The second generation, used in 1974 and 1975, had only one pump and expansile cylinders. However, the pump was difficult to handle, and deflation was painful for the patient. The cylinders, which were also hard to insert, tended to bulge out when inflated. Leaks occurred because of tube inlet wear or because of material fatigue. For the third model, implanted from 1975 to 1978, a pump that was slightly easier to deflate was developed. However, the all-silicone-rubber reservoir often leaked at its seams.

The fourth series first saw the seamless, dip-coated reservoir still used today, which is more reliable regarding leakage. The spherical shape provides it with higher mechanical stability and makes implantation easier. Furthermore, rear-tip extenders were developed, which facilitated the sizing of the cylinders and further reduced mechanical failures by allowing the cylinders to be more accurately positioned. Unfortunately, the devices still contained an internal reinforcing rod, which frequently led to wearing of the cylinder walls.

The development of the last generation, the so-called IPP 700, which has been available since 1983, clearly reduced mechanical failures, thanks to tremendous technical improvements, thus answering the problems that had been observed in previous models. Kinking of the tubes between pump and reservoir was prevented by a solid helix in the tube wall. The use of molding techniques lead to an easily reproducible pump, with a flat surface overlying the release valve, and with a smaller and clearly distinguishable layer between the valve and the surface of the control device. This made it easier for the patient to handle the device. In addition, the cylinder received a smoother, conical front tip, fitting better into the corpora cavernosa. On the other hand, the rear-tip extenders were made more blunt in order to prevent backward perforation through the wall of the crura. The expansive portion of the cylinder walls was made thicker in order to prevent bulging and to reduce leaks caused by material fatigue. Inlet tube wear was reduced by

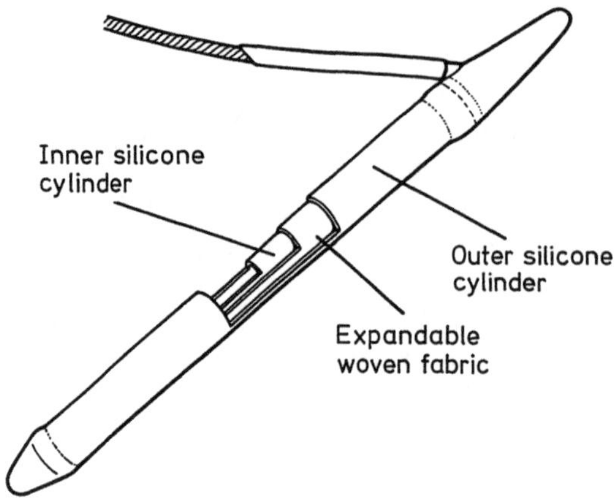

Fig. 2. The reinforced CX cylinder, which is more resistant against rupture and bulging than earlier generations (AMS Inservice)

covering the part of the tubes emerging from the cylinders with a more resistant nonabrasive coat. Last but not least, the reinforcing rod within the cylinder, which had led to wearing of the walls, was no longer used. Recently – in order to overcome cylinder bulging and rupture – a further improvement of the device was achieved: in the so-called CX cylinders, a textile layer was included within the silicone wall itself (Fig. 2). This will further reduce the incidence of cylinder leaks.

Throughout the evolution of the shape of the inflatable prosthesis, its operating principles basically remained the same. Erection is created in a quasi-natural way by pumping fluid, i.e., an isotonic saline solution with contrast medium, from a reservoir placed intraperitoneally or retropubically into two cylinders situated in the corpora cavernosa, all parts being connected by tubes. The filling of the expansive cylinders causes the penis to increase slightly in length and to a greater or lesser degree in circumference, depending on the thickness and the elasticity of the tunica albuginea. This erection is as close to normal as can be attained with a prosthesis. Deflation is obtained by pressing a metal valve in the control device, thus allowing the fluid to flow back into the reservoir. This control device, which integrates both pumping and the releasing mechanism, is placed in the scrotum. After being squeezed to complete the emptying of the cylinder, the penis hangs down in a fully natural position, in such a manner that the prosthesis is hardly noticed, even when the patient is undressed.

Another much-used fully inflatable device is the Mentor prosthesis, which is fundamentally an imitation of the IPP 700. It is made of a less elastic material called Bioflex, which makes this prosthesis less expansive. The deflation is also less marked, and therefore it cannot be worn as inconspicuously as the AMS model. On the other hand, the control device is easy to handle and not very susceptible to failure. All in all, there is little difference between this device and the IPP 700 (Engel et al. 1986; Merril and Javaheri 1984).

The latest development in inflatable penile devices is the so-called self-containing prosthesis. Basically, these devices operate in the same way as the fully inflatable ones, but they contain both the control mechanism and the fluid reservoir in the cylinder itself. The most important models are the Hydroflex (AMS) and the Flexiflate (Surgitek), both of which have the inflating pump in the tip of the cylinder. Squeezing this pump through the glans penis makes the saline solution shift from the reservoir into the central expansile chamber, and the penis stiffens. In the Hydroflex, the reservoir is in the rear tip, while in the Flexiflate it is in an outer space surrounding the expansive chamber. The Hydroflex is deflated by pressing a deflation valve behind the pumping device, and the Flexiflate by bending the penis downward firmly. The AMS device, therefore, has a slight advantage over the Flexiflate because incidental bending of the penis will not cause deflation, whereas this can occur in the Flexiflate. Undesired loss of erection during intercourse is reported frequently with the Flexiflate. Both devices have the functional and cosmetic disadvantage of poor deflation. Because of the small amount of fluid that is displaced, there is not much difference between erection and flaccidity. There is hardly any increase in circumference during erection, and after deflation, the penis remains in a semierect position. Furthermore, these devices contain an internal reinforcing rod, which increases the risk of backward migration or perforation that would lead to the so-called Concorde phenomenon – a drooping of the glans, no longer "armed", that makes intromission impossible. Due to these disadvantages, the self-containing devices do not offer much more comfort than the semirigid ones, but at a clearly higher price (Noll and Schreiter 1986; Schreiter 1985)!

Current Surgical Technique

The surgical approach can be infrapubic or penoscrotal. The subcoronal approach, proposed by many surgeons for semirigid implants, is not indicated for the hydraulic devices because of the postoperative danger of perforation. The perineal approach carries too much risk of infection. For the fully inflatable prosthesis, we prefer infrapubic implantation, which offers a lower infection rate and a reduced incidence of surgical failure; in addition, postoperative handling of the device is less painful for the patient. The self-containing models can be more easily implanted from a penoscrotal approach similar to that adopted for the semirigid models.

Which ever approach is chosen in prosthetic surgery, it is of the utmost importance to prevent perioperative infections. Therefore, the patient showers several hours before the operation, and his genital area is shaved immediately prior to surgery and washed again in the operating room with an antiseptic soap solution for about 15 min. In this way, hospital bacteria on the skin are eliminated.

The operation begins with a transverse infrapubic incision, the penis being stretched by the Scott retractor (Fig. 3). The tunica albuginea is incised longitudinally with a diathermic knife, and the corpora cavernosa are dilated with Hegar's dilators up to Hegar 13. The length and caliber of the corpus are measured using the scale on the Furlow inserter. The appropriate cylinder is then inserted, using the suture at its tip, which is attached to a straight needle loaded in the inserter. After the Furlow device has been inserted up to the cavernosal tip, the needle is pushed through the glans penis by means of the obturator. By pulling on the suture, the cylinder nose can be placed exactly in the tip of the cavernosal body

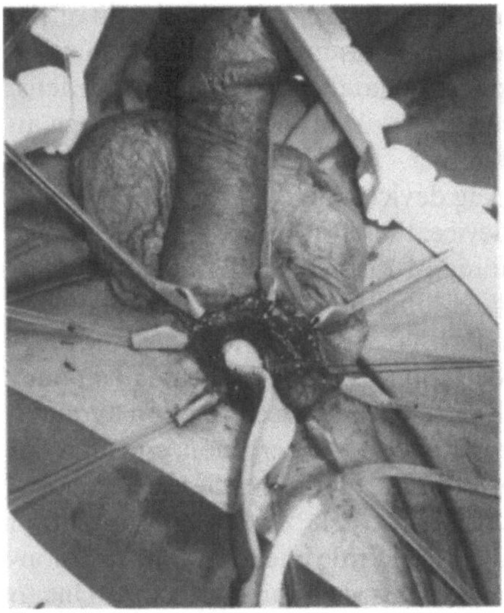

Fig. 3. The infrapubic approach, made using the Scott retractor. The cylinder is inserted by pulling on the suture previously pushed through the glans with the Furlow inserter

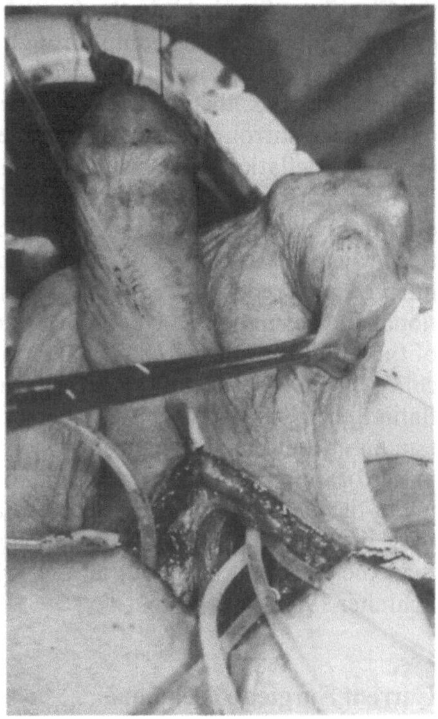

Fig. 4. The pump is placed in the scrotum

(Fig. 3). A rear-tip extender of the right size is then fitted onto the cylinder and inserted in the crus of the corpus cavernosum. Great care should be taken that the inlet tube leaves the cavernosal body without kinking. The tunica albuginea is closed with a running 3×0 monofilament resorbable suture, and the procedure is repeated on the other side. After the bladder has been emptied, the reservoir is inserted in the retropubic space or intraperitoneally and then filled. Via the same incision, the pump is placed in a space prepared between scrotal skin and the dartos layer (Fig. 4). After all the tubes have been connected the incision is closed by means of a running suture of both subcutaneous tissue and skin. No drain is left, in order to avoid infection (Fishmann et al. 1984; Furlow 1978; Noll/Schreiter 1986; Schreiter 1974; Schreiter et al. 1976).

Current Results

Since 1973, we have treated 235 patients in our department with an inflatable penile prosthesis. By May 1987, 191 patients had received the IPP 700, and 13 the Mentor inflatable; 21 patients were helped with the Hydroflex, and 10 with the Flexiflate. The age of these patients varied from 19 up to 74 years, most implantations being performed in men aged between 51 and 60 years. The main indication was diabetes mellitus (Table 1), followed by vascular disease, paraplegia, urethral injury, Peyronie's disease, radical prostatectomy or cystectomy, fibrosis

Table 1. Indications for implantation of hydraulic penile prostheses in 235 patients

Indication	No. of cases
Diabetes mellitus	46 (20%)
Vascular disease	35 (15%)
Paraplegia	27 (12%)
Urethral injury	24 (10%)
Peyronie's disease	23 (10%)
Radical prostatectomy	23 (10%)
Radical cystectomy	16 (7%)
Fibrosis after priapism	14 (6%)
Radical pelvic surgery	13 (6%)
Genital trauma	7 (3%)
Organic cause unknown	7 (3%)

Table 2. Surgical complications in 191 patients treated with AMS inflatable penile prostheses

Complication	Generation (no. of cases)			
	1–3	4 (RTE)	5 (IPP 700)	Total
Infection	2	3	2	9 (4%)
Tube kinking	2	2	0	4
Erosion	1	1	0	2
Hematoma	1	2	0	3
Pump malposition	0	1	0	1
Necrosis of corpora cavernosa	0	1	0	1
Cardiac arrest	0	1	0	1
Total	6/26 (23%)	11/52 (21%)	2/113 (2%)	21/191 (11%)

Table 3. Mechanical complications in 191 patients treated with AMS inflatable penile prostheses

Complication	Generation (no. of cases)			
	1–3	4 (RTE)	5 (IPP 700)	Total
Cylinder leakage	4	4	2	10 (5%)
Reservoir leakage	1	1	0	2
Connector leakage	2	1	0	3
Cylinder bulging	2	2	1	5
Malposition of cylinder	0	0	1	1
Total	9/26 (35%)	8/52 (15%)	4/113 (4%)	21/191 (11%)

after priapism, radical surgery of the pelvis for nonurological tumors, and genital traumata. In 3% of the men, no organic cause was found for the erectile dysfunction: they may have had psychogenic impotence. In the later series, we excluded patients of this kind from surgery because we believe that they are better off with sexual therapy.

We related all the surgical and mechanical complications that occurred in the 191 patients treated with the fully inflatable AMS prosthesis to the various generations of the device, as shown in Tables 2, 3. It is significant that the mechanical failure rate dropped from 35% for the first three generations to less than 4% for the IPP 700: this demonstrates spectacular improvements made in the device. However, the surgical complication rate was also reduced from 23% to 2% due to increasing experience and constant improvement of our surgical technique. The low infection rate overall is also very remarkable: it supports our opinion that perioperative antibiotics and meticulous antisepsis are extremely important.

In our series, the same favorable evolution can be seen in the incidence of correction of the devices (Table 4). While in the first three generations nearly 60% needed to be corrected (an incidence of about 0.5), we reduced the incidence of correction to one-tenth of this figure with the IPP 700 generation. The main com-

Table 4. Incidence of correction in five generations of AMS inflatable penile prostheses implanted in 191 patients

Generation	No. of corrections	Incidence
1–3 (1973–1977)	15/26	0.58
4 (RTE) (1978–1982)	19/52	0,37
5 (IPP 700) (1983–1987)	6/113	0.05

Table 5. Response of patients and partners to prosthetic implants

	Men	Women
Very satisfied	94 (81%)	78 (92%)
Satisfied	15 (13%)	3 (4%)
Not satisfied	7 (6%)	3 (4%)

Table 6. Reasons for dissatisfaction with prosthetic implants

	Men	Women
Length and rigidity	2	1
Loss of ejaculation	1	1
Pain	1	0
Loss of sensibility	1	0
Psychological problems	2	1
Total	7	3

plication leading to correction – leakage of the cylinders – was diminished to 2%, and this downward trend seems to be continuing with the new, reinforced CX cylinder. According to the first reports, covering more than 200 implantations performed by 46 surgeons, correction was required because of leakage in only 27 cases.

Our experience reveals a primary success rate of 95% for the IPP 700; after correction, the final success rate is 98%. Of the 191 men treated, 116 were interviewed, and 94% of them were at least satisfied with the prosthesis. Furthermore, 81 (96%) of the 84 women interviewed were satisfied with their partners' implants (Table 5). The main reasons for dissatisfaction are shown in Table 6 (Apte et al. 1984; Beutler et al. 1984; Gerstenberger et al. 1979; Malloy et al. 1986; Schreiter 1974, 1985; Schreiter et al. 1976; Scott et al. 1973, 1983).

Our experience with the other hydraulic devices is relatively limited and does not enable us to draw any conclusions. However, the Mentor device seems to produce good results like the IPP 700, albeit with slightly less satisfaction due to the less natural flaccidity. The self-containing prostheses need further development, especially as regards deflation. We do not consider them as our first choice, but if a patient, in full knowledge of their disadvantages, so wishes we do also implant these devices.

Conclusion

In summary, our 14 years of experience with the inflatable penile prosthesis have served to provide a large number of impotent men with a quasi-natural erection and physiological flaccidity; there has been a high degree of satisfaction on the part of both patients and their partners. Thanks to the continuous improvement of the devices and our increasing experience, both mechanical and surgical complications have decreased. The IPP 700 device (AMS) – especially with the new CX cylinders – answers all of the problems that have occurred with the previous models. We have implanted it in 113 patients, with only two mechanical and four surgical failures. We are convinced that an inflatable prosthesis provides the best functional and cosmetic way of restoring a lost erection, and one that is also very safe over a period of years. Further development, especially of the self-containing devices, will confirm prosthetic surgery as the most important treatment of erectile dysfunction in the near future.

References

Apte SM, Gregory JG, Purcell MH (1984) The inflatable penile prosthesis, reoperation and patient satisfaction. J Urol 131:894–895

Beutler LE, Scott FB, Karacan I, Baer PE, Royen RR, Morris J (1984) Women's satisfaction with partners' penile implant: inflatable vs. non inflatable. Urology 24:552

Engel RME, Smolev JK, Hackler R (1986) Experience with the Mentor inflatable penile prosthesis. J Urol 135:1181–1182

Finney RP (1977) New hinged silicone penile implant. J Urol 118:585

Finney RP (1984) Finney flexirod prosthesis. Urology 23:

Fishmann IJ, Scott FB, Light JK (1984) Experience with inflatable penile prosthesis. Urology 23:
Furlow WL (1978) Inflatable penile prosthesis: new device for cylinder insertion. Urology 12:447
Gerstenberger DL, Osborne D, Furlow WL (1979) Inflatable penile prosthesis, follow-up study of patient-partner satisfaction. Urology 12:583
Jonas U (1983) Five year's experiences with the silicone-silver prosthesis: improvements and new development. World J Urol 1:251
Jonas U, Jacobi GH (1980) Silicone-silver penile prosthesis. J Urol 123:865
Kothari DR, Timm GW, Frohrib DA, Bradley WE (1972) An implantable fluid transfer system for treatment of impotence. J Biomechan 5:567–570
Malloy TR, Wein AJ, Carpiniello VL (1980) Comparison of the inflatable penile and Small-Carrion prosthesis in the surgical treatment of erectile impotence. J Urol 123:678
Malloy TR, Wein A, Carpiniello V (1986) Reliability of AMS 700 inflatable penile prosthesis. Urology 28:385
Merril MD, Javaheri P (1984) Mentor inflatable penile prosthesis. Urology 23:46
Montague DK (1984) Experience with Jonas malleable penile prosthesis. Urology 23
Noll F, Schreiter F (1986) Erste Erfahrungen mit der AMS Hydroflex Penisprothese. Verh Dtsch Ges Urol 38:419
Porst H (1987) Erektile Impotenz. Enke
Schreiter F (1974) Die operative Behandlung der erektilen Impotenz mit Kunststoffprothesen. Aktuel Urol 5:95–99
Schreiter F (1985) Prothesenchirurgie des Penis. Angio Archiv 8:38–46
Schreiter F, Sholuda D, Bressel M (1976) Die chirurgische Behandlung der erektilen Dysfunktion mit der AMS-Penisprothese. Urology [A] 5:276–281
Scott FB, Bradley WE, Timm G (1973) Management of erectile impotence: use of implantable inflatable prosthesis. Urology 2:80
Scott FB, Fishmann IJ, Light JK (1983) A decade of experience with the inflatable penis prosthesis. World J Urol 1:244–250
Small MP (1984) Surgical treatment of impotence with Small Carrion prosthesis. Urology 23:8
Wespes E (1987) Impuissance organique masculine. Acta Urol Belg 55:141–330

The Use of Penile Prostheses in Impotence

L. V. Wagenknecht

Urology Clinic, Civic Hospital Cuxhaven, Altenwalder Chaussee 10–12, 2190 Cuxhaven, FRG

Thirty years ago, Couvelaire and Herlyn used ribs or parts of the tibia to reinforce the penis (see Wagenknecht et al. 1981; Wagenknecht 1987). Between 1960 and 1970, unilateral penile prostheses were used (Pearman, Lash-Loeffler, and Tudoriu, in Wagenknecht et al. 1981). Because of the penile anatomy, these devices could not be implanted in between the corpora cavernosa, but entered one or other of the corpora. Lesions and penetration of the urethra, glans, and crura penis were frequent. Rigid double prostheses were developed in 1965 by El-Masri and in 1966 by Beheri (Wagenknecht et al. 1981; Wagenknecht 1987). Tudoriu proposed a fork-shaped Teflon prosthesis to be implanted under Buck's fascia over the corpora cavernosa. The Small-Carrion silicone double prosthesis proved to be the most widely used penile prosthesis for more than 12 years (Carrion 1986). This prosthesis was implanted in 50000 men, with a complication rate of only 3%–5% (Carrion 1986).

There are two kinds of flexible silicone penile prostheses: the Subrini design (Fig. 1), with two different segments of silicone and a proximal segment for shortening of the device and the Finney implant, with proximal segments for shortening to individual requirements (Finney et al. 1980; Subrini 1980; Wagenknecht et al. 1981). Following implantation of these prostheses, the penis is supposed to hang loosely in a normal position; however, buckling may occur. In 1975, Tudoriu proposed a flexible prosthesis, which was successfully employed by the author in over 300 men (Wagenknecht et al. 1981).

Malleable penile prostheses such as the Jonas device (Fig. 2), the AMS Malleable 600 (Fig. 3), and the Mentor Malleable consist of a silicone cylinder with an inner metal band, which permits malleability in every direction and is sup-

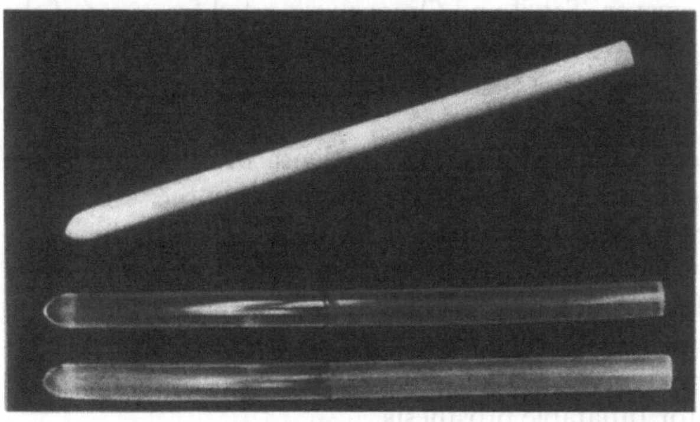

Fig. 1. Subrini penile prosthesis

Plastic Surgery in the Sexually Handicapped
Eds.: W. Eicher/Kubli/Herms

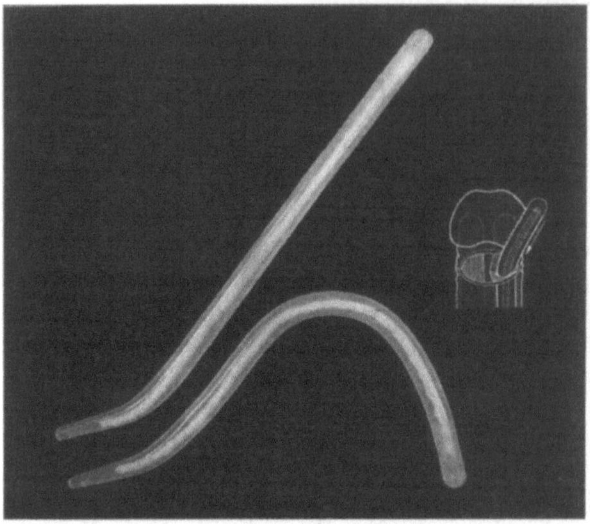

Fig. 2. Jonas penile prosthesis

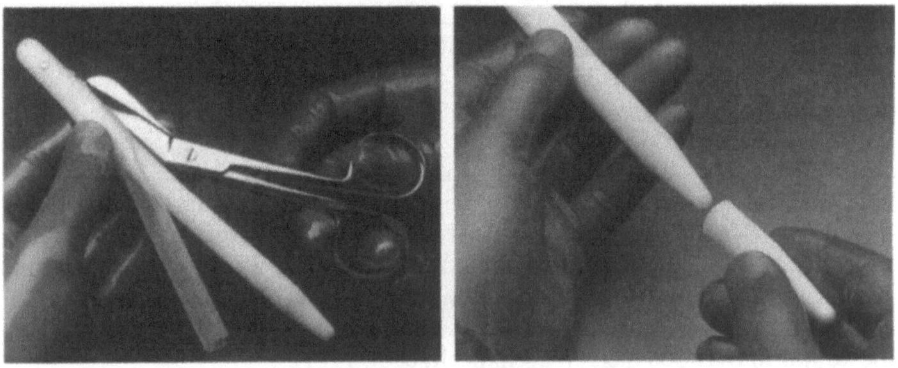

Fig. 3. AMS Malleable 600 penile prosthesis

posed to resist breaking. However, Tawil and Gregory reported fractures of the Jonas silver wire in 7 of 23 cases (Wagenknecht 1988). Malleable penile prostheses are a good compromise, with reasonable costs, short hospitalization, and few mechanical problems or complications.

Hydraulic penile prostheses were first described by Scott, Bradley, and Timm in 1973 (for details, see Wagenknecht et al. 1981): a pump within the scrotum allows fluid to be shifted from a reservoir behind the rectus muscle into the inflatable double cylinders within the corpora cavernosa (Fig. 4). The one-way valves of this system allow simulated erection to be maintained for the desired time, and a separate backflow mechanism is initiated via a valve in the scrotum for deflation. The best hydraulic penile prostheses currently on the market are the AMS Inflatable 700 and the Mentor Inflatable prosthesis.

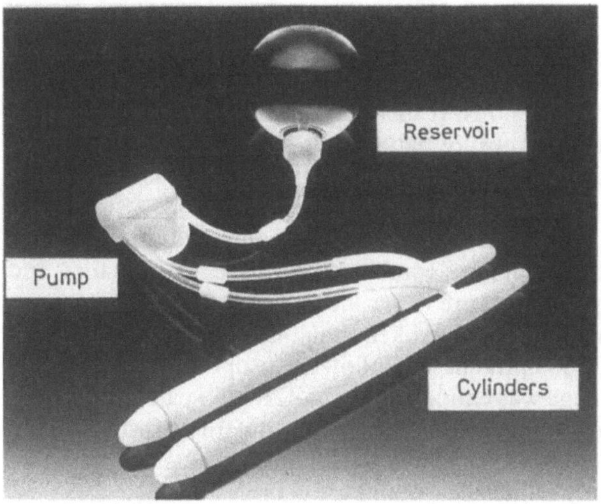

Fig. 4. AMS Inflatable 700 penile prosthesis

Recent new developments (the AMS Hydroflex and Surgitek Flexiflate) can be implanted like rod prostheses in both corpora cavernosa. Within the stable proximal portion, they contain fluid, which is shifted for "erection" into the anterior inflatable chamber by manipulating a pump device behind the glans. These prostheses are being tested clinically at the moment.

Indications

The indications for penile prostheses are as follows (Table 1):

1. Diabetes mellitus
2. Arterial lesions with diminished blood flow
3. Combined venous leakage factors
4. Combined arteriovenous insufficiency
5. Fibrosis of the corpora cavernosa after priapism
6. After penile trauma
7. Penile induration (Peyronie's disease)
8. Lesions of the lumbar spine and of pelvic nerves
9. After pelvic fracture with urethral rupture
10. After operations in the lower pelvis (e.g., radical prostatectomy or rectum amputation)
11. After perineal operations (e.g., urethral plastics).

The surgical approach for implantation of rod prostheses may involve (a) dorsal incision behind the glans, (b) perineal incision, (c) penile shaft incision, (d) penoscrotal incision, and (e) infrapubic, presymphyseal incision. We prefer the infrapubic appraoch; however, a circumcision approach is prefered if there is a short frenulum or phimosis.

Results

Table 1 shows the various operations performed in our institution over a period of 3.5 years for different erectile lesions. It includes details of various treatment modalities used for different subgroups of patients.

In 100 patients, the following penile prostheses were used: 20 Small-Carrion devices, 33 Jonas silver-wire prostheses, 2 Subrini implants, and 45 malleable AMS prostheses (Figs. 1–4). The main indications were combined arteriovenous insufficiency, leakage from the albuginea, combined venous leakage factors, and reduced arterial flow. In 95 patients, there was a successful postoperative course, with no complications. In one patient, a broken Small-Carrion implant was replaced with a malleable AMS 600 prosthesis. Following a suprapubic hematoma in two patients, suction drainage was employed for 24 h. In two patients with extensive penile induration, the implantation of the penile prosthesis was difficult, and the device had to be covered with a rectus-fascia flap. Two patients presented a slightly diminished sensitivity of the skin behind the glans following a dorsal incision there.

Infectious complications in five patients required removal of the prosthesis. In one of these patients, partial amputation of the penis was necessary following five separate interventions for drainage of abscesses. Three of the five failures occurred in diabetics, in whom prevention of infection is particularly important. The necessary measures to this end include: (a) aminoglycoside antibiosis

Table 1. Surgical treatment in 217 patients presenting various erectile lesions

Erectile lesion	Surgery	No. of cases	Results	
			Good	Bad
Penile deviation	Cavernous wedge incision (Nesbit procedure; dorsal 21, ventral 3)	24	24	0
Penile induration	Cavernous wedge incision	3	2	1
	Cavernous cylinder excision	6	5	1
	Penile prosthesis	10	10	0
Penile trauma	Reconstruction	12	12	0
	Penile prosthesis	4	4	0
Fibrosis after priapism	Ligation of shunt	4	2	2
	Penile prosthesis	18	17	1
Leakage factor	Vein ligation	52	36	16
	Penile prosthesis	13	13	0
Decreased blood flow	Arterialization of penile vein	10	8	2
	Penile prosthesis	28	26	2
Arteriovenous insufficiency	Arterialization and vein ligation	4	2	2
	Penile prosthesis	27	25	2
Total		217	186	31

(3 × 80 mg for 8–10 days, starting 24 h prior to operation), (b) shaving of the genital area 24–48 h prior to the intervention, (c) antiseptic baths before operation, (d) careful and repeated disinfection of the wound area during operation, and (e) change of gloves prior to implantation of the prosthesis.

Discussion

The advantages and disadvantages of penile prostheses are as follows. Rod prostheses are easy to implant, can be obtained at a reasonable price, require short postoperative hospitalization, and have a low complication rate (2%–5%). A disadvantage is the permanent erection they produce, which may become noticeable under certain types of clothing. Cystoscopy is possible and should be performed with flexible instruments. Transurethral resection may be done via a perineal urethrotomy (boutonniere). Perforations caused by rod prostheses have been described (Gasser et al., cited in Wagenknecht 1988). We prefer the AMS Malleable 600 (Fig. 3): 3 pairs of prostheses are sufficient for 12 different lenghts (proximal tip extenders) and for 2 different calibers (removable silicone sheath).

Hydraulic penile prostheses offer the advantage of best simulating the mechanism of erection and deflation. The AMS Inflatable 700 best guarantees sufficient penile rigidity for sexual intercourse and physiologic deflation. The Mentor Inflatable also seems to be of appropriate quality (see F. Schreiter and J. Denil, this volume). The disadvantages of the hydraulic prostheses are (a) the relatively complicated operative technique; (b) mechanical problems requiring reparative interventions (Leaks in the fluid reservoir or the valves, kinking of the tubes); (c) the long operation and hospitalization; and (d) the high cost of the prostheses. The overall complication rate decreased from 22% 5 years ago to 5%–10% nowadays (Furlow 1986; Schreiter 1987; Wagenknecht et al. 1981). For details about the various prostheses, the reader is referred to the manufacturers' information and to the medical literature (Furlow, Tudoriu, Small, Kelâmi, Finney, Jonas, Raz, Boxer, Kaufman, Hasche-Klünder, cited in Wagenknecht et al. 1981).

Implantation of a penile prosthesis has to be the last of a series of treatment modalities. Psychosomatic cooperation is required in order to avoid implant-related psychopathology. The advantages and particularly the disadvantages have to be discussed with both husband and wife. One should not raise more hopes than the prosthesis can fulfill.

References

Carrion HM (1988) Results of 50000 Small-Carrion implants. Proc Androl Symp Rome 1986 (in press)

Finney RP, Sharpe JR, Sadlowski RW (1980) Finney hinged penile implant: experience with 100 cases. J Urol 124:205–207

Furlow WL (1986) Implantation of the inflatable penile prosthesis Model AS 700: current results and long-term follow-up. Proceedings of the 2nd World Congress on Impotence, University Press Prague

Jonas V (1987) Development and indication of penile prosthesis in the treatment of erectile dysfunction. Proceedings of the 10th International Symposium of the Medical Academy of Vienna, Academy Press, Vienna

Schreiter F (1987) Hydraulic prostheses AMS 700 and AMS Hydroflex. Proceedings of the Symposium on Prostheses in Urology, Masson Lyon

Subrini L (1980) Treatment of impotence using penile implants. In: Forleo R, Pasini W (eds) Medical Sexology. 3. Int. Cong., Amsterdam

Wagenknecht LV, Furlow WL, Auvert J (1981) Urogenital reconstruction with prostheses. Thieme, Stuttgart

Wagenknecht LV (1988) Impotenz: Pathophysiologie, Diagnostik, Therapie. Diesbach, Berlin

Part 7: Vascular Impotence

Treatment of Vasculogenic Impotence

V. Michal and T. Klika

Institute for Clinical Experimental Medicine, Cardiovascular Research Programme, Vídenská 800, PO Box 10, 14000 Prague 4, Czechoslovakia

Impotence, together with arterial disease, is one of the most frequent affections of middle-aged and elderly men. Available data indicate that the incidence of impotence is nearly twice as high as that of ischemic heart disease, and both conditions are similarly age dependent.

A high incidence of stenoses and occlusions of the arterial bed supplying the corpora cavernosa was documented 11 years ago in patients suffering from impotence by means of arteriographic techniques developed by J. F. Ginestié and also in our institute.

We used artificial erection induced by intracavernous infusion of heparinized saline, originally as an adjuvant method in phalloarteriography. Together with intracavernous administration of papaverine and monitoring of intracavernous pressure, circumferential changes, and infusion rates, this became a type of functional examination of the corpora cavernosa able to answer the basic questions concerning the hemodynamics of erection.

The process can be subdivided into two stages: in the first one, the arterial system must deliver to the corpora cavernosa at least a threshold volume (approx. 140 ml) and provide a minimum pressure (over 65 mmHg) to fill and distend them. In the second stage, the corpora cavernosa function as a closed system. Contractions of the ischiocavernous muscles compress the crura in their osteomuscular channels and increase intracavernous pressure to suprasystolic values (150–250 mmHg, with peaks exceeding 400 mmHg).

In 62 patients with severe erectile disorders, examination showed normal hemodynamics of erection in 11 (18%), insufficient inflow in 21 (34%), insufficient blockage of outflow in 14 (22.5%), and a combination of both of the latter in 15 (24%). Insufficient contraction of ischio cavernous muscles alone was found in one patient with polyradiculoneuritis and was also found in combination with other insufficiencies (partially as a consequence of these) in a further 10 patients.

Intracavernous injection of papaverine and α-blockers is effective in psychogenic and neurogenic impotence, but only in milder forms of vasculogenic impotence. In all these cases, maximal vasodilatation of the afferent arterial bed and maximal relaxation of smooth muscles inside the corpora cavernosa are able to compensate for relative insufficiency of the arterial bed and reduced blockage of venous drainage.

Vascular surgery can either restore and increase arterial inflow by reconstruction of the affected bed supplying the erectile bodies or decrease venous drainage by occlusion of the draining veins; finally, it can affect both of these components

Plastic Surgery in the Sexually Handicapped
Eds.: W. Eicher/Kubli/Herms

to a greater or lesser degree by construction of arteriovenous or arteriocavernous shunts or a combination of these.

A total of 322 vascular operations for erectile disorders have been performed at our Institute. (This number does not include 42 arteriocavernous shunts performed between 1973 and 1979.) The indications for these operations were based on the examination of pressure in penile arteries, arteriography, and phalloarteriography; since 1983, functional examination of the corpora cavernosa by means of artificial erection and, in some cases, cavernosography have also been performed.

The arterial bed supplying the erectile bodies comprises the arteries of the aortoiliac area, the hypogastric, internal pudendal, penile, bulbourethral, dorsal, and deep penile arteries. From the technical point of view, the indication for reconstruction of this bed is determined by the type and location of the lesions and by the accessibility of the different arterial segments.

In aortoiliac occlusive disease, improvement of arterial flow to the corpora cavernosa can be a by-product of aortoiliac reconstruction, and the treatment should include reconstruction of the hypogastric arteries. Isolated lesions of the hypogastric arteries have been managed by percutaneous transluminal angioplasty, by iliacohypogastric venous bypass, or by open endarterectomy. The middle part of the internal pudendal artery can be reached by the gluteal approach and, depending on the arteriographic findings, an iliaco- or gluteopudendal bypass can be constructed. The distal part of the internal pudendal artery is approached by a perineal incision and femoropudendal autovenous bypass was the first procedure we used for reconstruction of this bed in 1972.

The whole proximal part of the arterial bed supplying the corpora cavernosa can be bypassed by end-to-side epigastricopenile anastomosis which we started to use in 1977. This procedure is indicated in those cases in which the branching of the penile artery remains patent and the deep penile and accessory deep penile arteries and the corpora cavernosa can be supplied by backflow.

Of the patients operated on, 74% were satisfied with the outcome; this was occasionally confirmed by their sexual partners. The best results were achieved with reconstruction of the hypogastric arteries: 80% of the patients completely regained erectility. The lower success rate of microvascular procedures could be explained by the lower patency rate. However, 13 patients who underwent microvascular procedures and 20 who underwent reconstruction of the hypogastric arteries reported little or no improvement despite patent reconstructions. This was probably due to further peripheral lesions or to unrecognized further factors, e.g., leakage from the corpora cavernosa. After surgery, three recent patients preoperatively unresponsive to intracavernous administration of 60 mg papaverine got full erections after administration of only 5 mg. Two of these patients became independent of these injections after five and seven applications, respectively.

Ligature of the deep dorsal vein or its varicose branches was indicated in 16 patients who showed symptoms of inadequate blockage of venous drainage during functional examination. In three patients, we ligated the varicose veins perforating the tunica albuginea, and the openings in the tunica could be sutured. While improvement of erectility lasting for 6 months after the operation was recorded in 11 patients (67%), it lasted longer than 1 year in only 7 (44%), these results suggest gradual restoration of increased drainage.

Construction of arteriovenous shunts was introduced into the surgery of impotence by Le Veen in 1980. It takes the form of a bypass from the femoral artery to the deep dorsal vein or anastomosis of the epigastric artery to this vein. The aim of the procedure is to increase pressure in the penile venous system and improve blockage of venous outflow during erection. Virag modified arterialization of the deep dorsal vein by central ligature of this vein. Further increase of the pressure in the venous system reverses the flow in the deep dorsal vein and may also ensure retrograd filling of the corpora cavernosa during erection. Peripheral ligature can prevent congestion in the glans and corpus spongiosum of the urethra, which represents an unpleasant complication of arterialization.

These types of procedures were performed in 15 patients who showed abnormal leakage from the corpora cavernosa during the functional examination and/or peripheral arterial lesions which could hardly be managed by reconstruction. The procedures resulted in the resumption of sexual life by 11 patients (73%); however, the good result only lasted longer than 1 year in 9 of them.

To summarize, our results have shown that vascular and microvascular surgery can correct at least some of the defects in the hemodynamics of erection and restore natural erections in the majority of patients operated on. Refinement of our differential diagnostic and microsurgical techniques and more experience of indications could further improve the success rate of these procedures, whose basic advantage is the restoration of natural erections.

Arterialization Techniques for Impotence

L. V. Wagenknecht

Urology Clinic, Civic Hospital, 2190 Cuxhaven, FRG

The arterial network of the penis is demonstrated in Fig. 1. Microsurgical revascularization of the penis was first described by Michal et al. in 1973 as an anastomosis between the superficial epigastric artery and the corpus cavernosum. The pioneers of penile revascularization, Michal, Ginestie, Crespo, Zorgniotti, Hauri, and Virag, used the superior and inferior epigastric artery and saphenous vein grafts for anastomoses to the corpus cavernosum and to the dorsal penile artery, with and without anastomoses to the penile dorsal vein (Figs. 2, 3). The early suc-

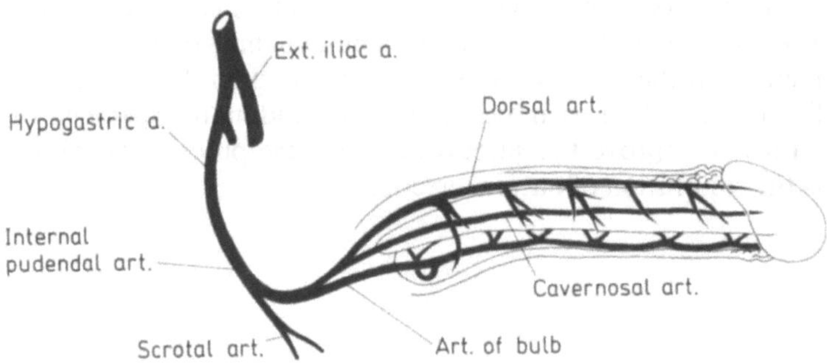

Fig. 1. Arterial supply of the penis

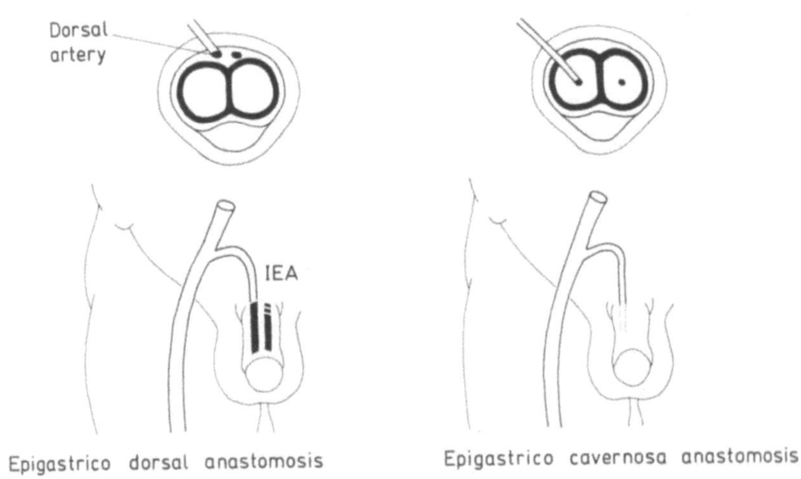

Fig. 2. Early arterialization techniques. *IEA,* inferior epigastric artery. (From Porst 1988)

Plastic Surgery in the Sexually Handicapped
Eds.: W. Eicher/Kubli/Herms

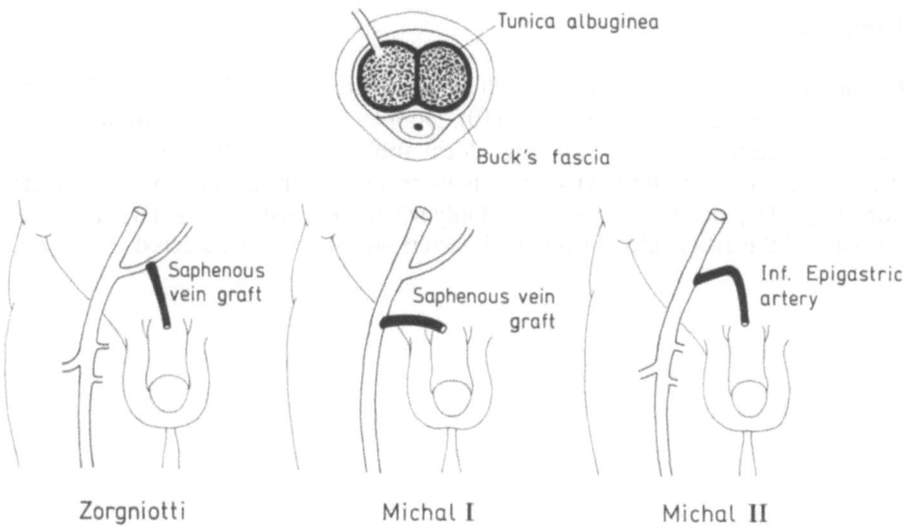

Fig. 3. Various grafts for penile arterialization. (From Porst 1988)

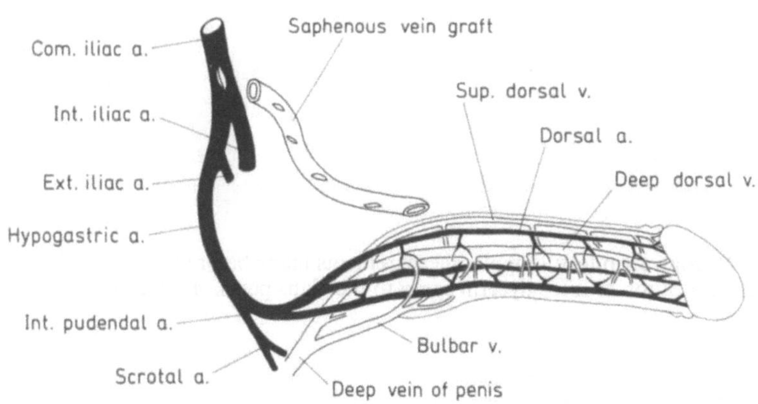

Fig. 4. Interposition of saphenous vein graft between common iliac artery and deep dorsal penile vein

cess rate for these procedures ranged between 40% and 90% (Michal et al. 1986; Ginestie and Romieux 1978; Crespo et al. 1986; Zorgniotti and Rossi 1985; Hauri 1987; Virag 1984). Anastomoses between epigastric artery and dorsal penile artery functioned well 3 years later in 20%–60% (Michal et al. 1986; Crespo et al. 1986; Zorgniotti and Rossi 1985; Hauri 1987; Virag 1984; Sarramon 1985). In 1982, because of the mediocre results of the latter procedures, Virag proposed interposition of the saphenous vein between iliac artery and deep dorsal penile vein. We have adopted this method because it offers higher flow rates than other procedures (Fig. 4). First results and intraoperative modifications will be presented below.

Diagnosis

During the last 4 years, more than 300 patients with erectile disorders underwent a staged diagnosis in our institution (10). Doppler flowmetry was combined with the nitroglycerin test: before and after local application of nitroglycerin spray to the glans penis, Doppler measurements were done over various portions of the dorsal and deep penile artery (Fig. 5). Only when these tests revealed a functional decrease of the article blood flow phalloarteriography was considered. However,

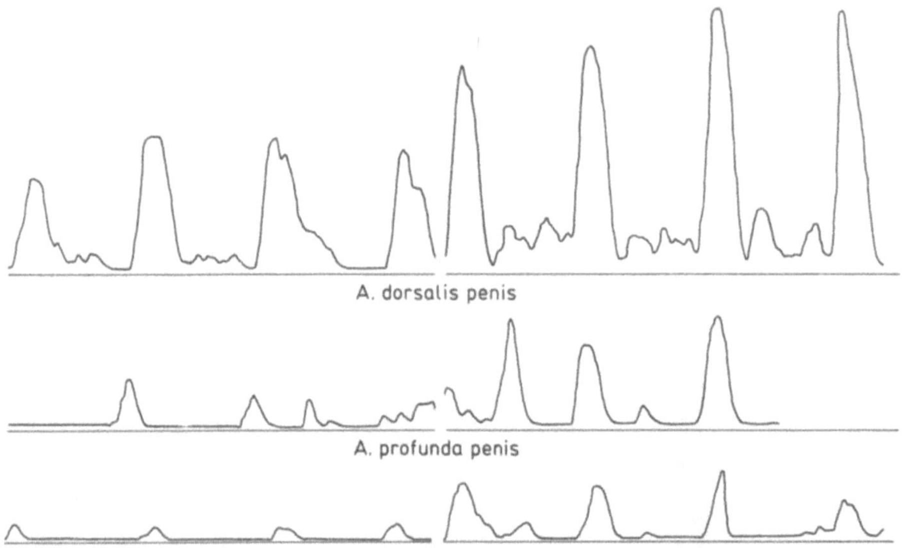

Fig. 5. Results of Nitroglycerin test: Doppler measurements made before (*left*) and 15 min after (*right*) local application of nitroglycerin spray to the glans penis. *A*, arteria

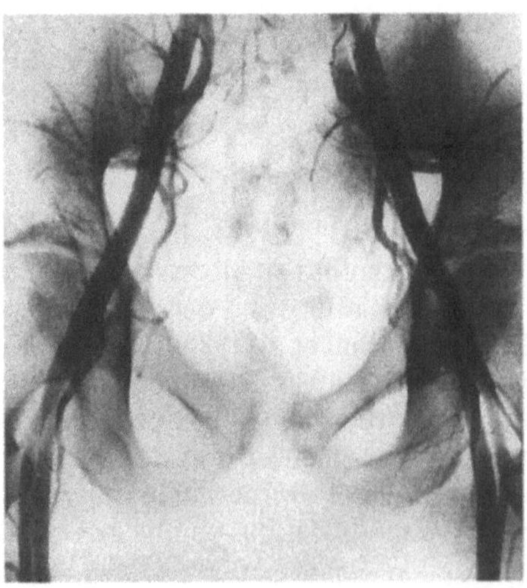

Fig. 6. Penile arteriogram: anteroposterior view demonstrates blockage of pudendal arteries

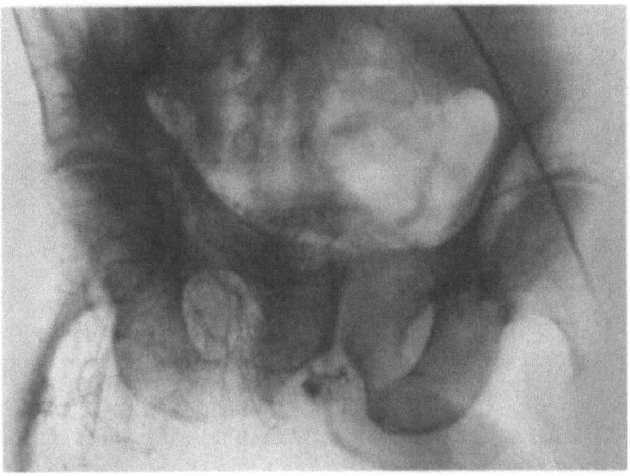

Fig. 7. Selective phalloarteriography: oblique view shows blockage of the dorsal penile artery, a patent cavernosal artery, and poor visualization of the deep penile artery

if dynamic cavernosography and cavernosometry in these patients showed an additional leakage factor which appeared not to be correctable by surgery, arteriography was abandoned, and penile prostheses were proposed. In the remaining patients, penile arteriography was done (Ginestie and Romieux 1978; Zorgniotti and Rossi 1985; Wagenknecht 1988; Figs. 6, 7). It is necessary to perform phlebography of the legs before considering use of the saphenous vein in order to determine the permeability of the deep veins for postoperative venous drainage.

Surgery

The operation is shown schematically in Fig. 4. Microsurgical qualifications and instruments are needed. Loupes of 4.5 × 6 magnification are used in combination with headlamps. Three incisions are necessary. After incision at the penile base and over the saphenous vein, lidocaine (Xylocaine) is injected around the vessels to prevent vasoconstriction. In preparing the saphenous vein, one should aim to use the longest possible portion of the vessel. Its lower end is brought to the freed iliac artery for the upper anastomosis in order to minimize the effect of the valves. Careful dilation of the vessel can be done with lidocaine irrigation. Instrumental dilation or incision of the valves damages the endothelium and increases the risk of later thromboses. Depending on the length of the saphenous vein, the common iliac artery or the external iliac artery is chosen for the anastomosis. If preoperative cavernosography demonstrated increased venous drainage, ligation of the internal iliac vein and of collaterals at the penile base may be necessary at this stage. Following prepubic transposition of the saphenous vein to the penile base, the deep dorsal vein is dissected, opened longitudinally, and anastomosed to the graft with 6 × 0 Prolene (Fig. 8). All patients were given heparin sodium (7500 IU/24 h) for 3 months. During surgery, the Depot-anti-androgen cyproterone acetate (Androcur, Schering, FRG) was given to prevent postoperative erections. Because of priapism in one case, we modified the surgical procedure. Artificial erec-

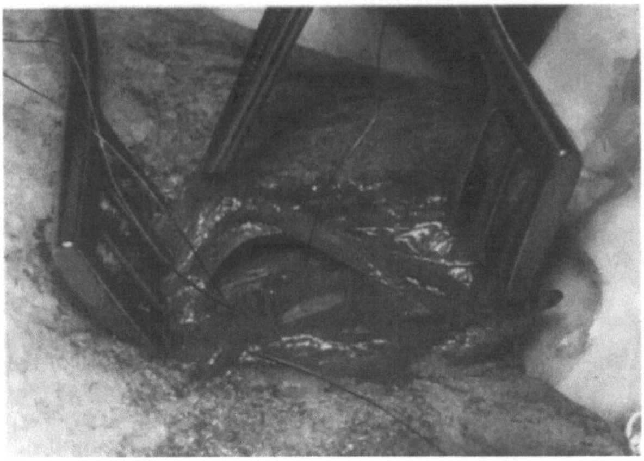

Fig. 8. Microsurgical anastomosis between saphenous vein graft and deep dorsal penile vein

tion and maintenance flow are measured (after ligation of venous collaterals for increased drainage). This maintenance flow is then correlated with the flow measurement of the saphenous graft (Fig. 4). The graft flow ranges between 40 and 120 ml/min. A calibrated roller infusion pump is used. In case of lower flow rates which do not match the maintenance flow of an artificial erection, the lower end of the saphenous vein graft is shortened. This increases the diameter of the vessel and allows a higher flow rate. The shortening of the graft may require an anastomosis to the *external* iliac artery instead of the common iliac artery.

Results

Of 300 patients with erectile lesions, Doppler flowmetry in combination with the nitroglycerin test showed a decreased arterial penile blood flow in 42. Dynamic cavernosography and cavernosometry demonstrated a concomitant increase of venous drainage in 38 of these men. Phalloarteriography was done in 22 patients and showed arteriosclerotic stenosis or traumatic occlusion of the internal pudendal artery in 21 of them. In 15 patients with an average age of 57, arterialization was done using a saphenous graft of 25–30 cm (Table 1). One patient developed priapism requiring ligation of the shunt. The average follow-up of the remaining 14 patients was 26 months. Doppler controls were done at 2- to 7-day intervals (Fig. 5). Excellent results were obtained in four patients presenting with traumatic occlusion of the internal pudendal artery. They all resumed full sexual activity 5–6 weeks postoperatively. Six further patients in the 5th decade of life presenting arteriosclerotic stenosis of the internal pudendal artery all showed good immediate results; 2 years later, four of them had open shunts and satisfactory potency. Two failures in this group coincided with diabetes mellitus. Combined arteriovenous insufficiency in four patients required additional ligation of venous collaterals at the penile base and ligation of both internal iliac veins. Two failures in this group also coincided with diabetes mellitus. Table 2 shows the frequency of penile arterialization as compared with other treatment modalities.

Table 1. Results of penile arterialization performed in 15 patients using a saphenous vein graft

Erectile lesion	No. of cases	Success		Failure
		After 1 month	After 2 years	
Traumatic occlusion of internal pudendal artery	4	4	4	0
Arteriosclerotic stenosis of internal pudendal artery	7	6	4	3
Arteriovenous insufficiency	4	2	2	2
Total	15	12	10	5

Table 2. Surgical treatment in 217 patients presenting various erectile lesions

Erectile lesion	Surgery	No. of cases	Results	
			Good	Bad
Penile deviation	Cavernous wedge, incision (Nesbit procedure; dorsal 21, ventral 3)	24	24	0
Penile induration	Cavernous wedge incision	3	2	1
	Cavernous cylinder excision	6	5	1
	Penile prosthesis	10	10	0
Penile trauma	Reconstruction	12	12	0
	Penile prosthesis	4	4	0
Fibrosis after priapism	Ligation of shunt	4	2	2
	Penile prosthesis	18	17	1
Leakage factor	Vein ligation	52	36	16
	Penile prosthesis	13	13	0
Decreased blood flow	Arterialization of penile vein	10	8	2
	Penile prosthesis	28	26	2
Arteriovenous insufficiency	Arterialisation and vein ligation	4	2	2
	Penile prosthesis	27	25	2
Total		217	186	31

One man presenting priapism after arterialization is not included.

Discussion

An exact diagnosis of the causes of impotence is the fundamental basis for the choice of treatment, and it can only be achieved by psychosomatic cooperation between various medical specialities. With the exception of phalloarteriography, the diagnostic sequence of investigations is noninvasive. A functional evaluation of penile arteries at the penile base, midshaft, and behind the glans can be done over the dorsal and deep penile artery with Doppler flowmetry. The nitroglycerin test allows to evaluate the vascular reaction: usually, one picks up higher Doppler waves, or there is a clear registration where no waves could be registered before. The combination of Doppler flowmetry and high-resolution ultrasound may also make arteriography unnecessary (Lue 1986). However, arteriography is needed before penile revascularization to locate the site of an obstruction (Michal et al. 1973, 1986; Ginestie and Romieux 1978; Crespo et al. 1986; Zorgniotti and Rossi 1985; Hauri 1987; Virag 1984; Sarramon 1985; Wagenknecht 1988; Virag 1986). Cavernosography and determination of the maintenance flow of an artificial erection are required to detect an additional leakage factor. The combined diagnostic investigations determine the indications for various procedures (Table 2). In well-selected cases, penile arterialization seems to be a logical treatment modality (Table 1).

Flow rates in the epigastric artery range between 20 and 40 ml/min, and those in a saphenous graft vary between 40 and 120 ml/min. We feel that the choice of shunt should be correlated with the flow rate necessary to maintain an artificial erection. Shortening the lower end of the saphenous vein increases the diameter of the graft and its flow rate. Lidocaine irrigation prevents vasoconstriction and helps to dilate the vessel. Virag reported a 3-year success rate of 70% after penile arterialization using a saphenous vein graft (1986). We feel that diabetics with pronounced neurovascular lesions are not suitable candidates for this procedure. Exact diagnosis and selection of patients with traumatic and arteriosclerotic occlusion of the internal pudendal artery is as important for postoperative success as the microsurgical technique.

References

Crespo EL, Bove D, Farrell G, Soltanik M (1986) Bypass permeability follow-up in 257 operated patients with our original microsurgical technique. Proceedings of the 2nd World Meeting on Impotence, Prague, 1986, University Press, Prague

Ginestie JF, Romieux A (1978) L'exploration radiologique de l'impuissance. Malonie, Paris

Hauri D (1987) Penile revascularisation. Proceedings of the 10th International Symposium, Vienna

Lue TF (1986) Functional evaluation of penile arteries with duplex-pulsed Doppler-analysis and high-resolution ultrasound. Proceedings of the 2nd World Meeting on Impotence, Prague, 1986, University Press, Prague

Michal V, Kramár R, Pospichal J, Hejhal L (1973) Prima tepenna anastomoza na corpora cavernosa penis v. lecbe erectivini impotence. Rozhl Chir 52:587

Michal V, Krysl J, Klika T, Fara P (1986) Revascularisation of the cavernous bodies. Proceedings of the 2nd World Meeting on Impotence. Prague, 1986, University Press, Prague

Porst H (1988) Erektile Impotenz. Enke, Stuttgart

Sarramon JP (1985) Penile revascularisation. In: Wagenknecht LV (ed) Microsurgery in Urology. Thieme-Stratton, New York

Virag R (1984) The treatment of angiogenic impotence. Int Angiol 3:275

Virag R (1986) Treatment of vascular impotence. Proceedings of the 2nd World Meeting on Impotence. Prague, 1986, University Press, Prague

Wagenknecht LV (1988) Impotenz: Pathophysiologie – Diagnostik – Therapie. Diesbach, Berlin

Zorgniotti AW, Rossi G (1985) Vasculogenic impotence. Thomas, Springfield

Therapy for Increased Venous Drainage in Organic Impotence

L. V. Wagenknecht

Urology Clinic, Civic Hospital, 2190 Cuxhaven, FRG

Increased drainage from the corpora cavernosa hinders the erectile high-pressure system (Lue et al. 1983). Recent results of dynamic cavernosograms, measurements of intracavernous pressure, and the maintenance index of erection have shown that various leaks may exist alone or in conjunction with other lesions (Lue et al. 1983; Buvat et al. 1986; Lewis et al. 1986; Stief 1986; Porst and Ahlen 1986; Virag 1985; Wespes and Schulman 1985; Wagenknecht and Shukfeh 1986). Increased venous drainage is diagnosed on the basis of early and later camera exposures during cavernosography, glans appearance time, and maintenance index. If a maintenance flow of more than 100–140 ml/min is necessary for erection, a leak may be assumed to exist.

Based on experience with 300 dynamic cavernosograms, details and illustrations of the following leakage factors were given elsewhere (Wagenknecht 1987): (a) single venous shunt, (b) traumatic leakage from the corpus spongiosum, (c) persisting shunt after surgery for priapism, (d) collateral veins to the saphenous and femoral veins, (e) penile induration with venous collaterals, (f) leakage to the glans penis and to the corpus spongiosum, and (g) combined arteriovenous insufficiency. Around the turn of the century, ligation of the dorsal penile vein was suggested by Duncan (1895), Wooten (1902), and Lydston (1908). In recent years, success rates of 10%–85% have been reported following ligation of the dorsal penile vein (Buvat et al. 1986; Lewis et al. 1986; Stief 1986; Wespes and Schulman 1985).

Methods

The venous system of the penis is shown in Fig. 1. Details of its anatomy and function are known (Lue et al. 1983; Lewis et al. 1986; Porst and Ahlen 1986; Wagenknecht 1984). Venous drainage of the corpora cavernosa occurs not only at the penile dorsum but also at the crura penis into the pudendal plexus and via collaterals to the saphenous and femoral vein (Fig. 2).

While venous collaterals to the saphenous and femoral vein may be ligated from an incision at the penile base, the branches to the epigastric and pudendal plexus cannot be reached from there. Since the internal iliac vein constitutes the confluent of the periprostatic and pudendal plexus, ligation of both internal iliac veins seems to be a logical consequence in cases of increased drainage via these vessels (Fig. 2).

Plastic Surgery in the Sexually Handicapped
Eds.: W. Eicher/Kubli/Herms

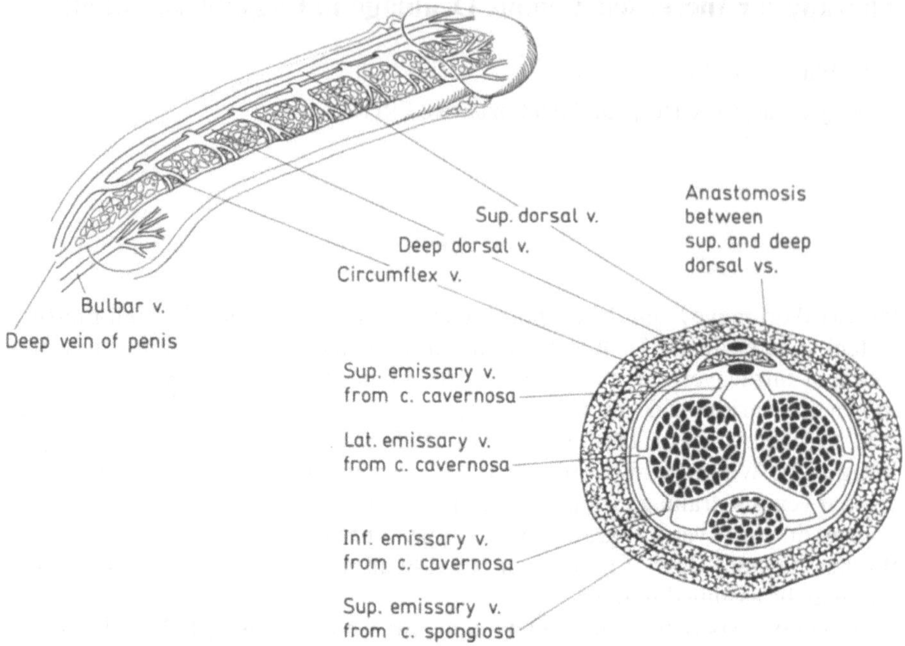

Fig. 1. Venous drainage of the penis. (From Rivard 1982)

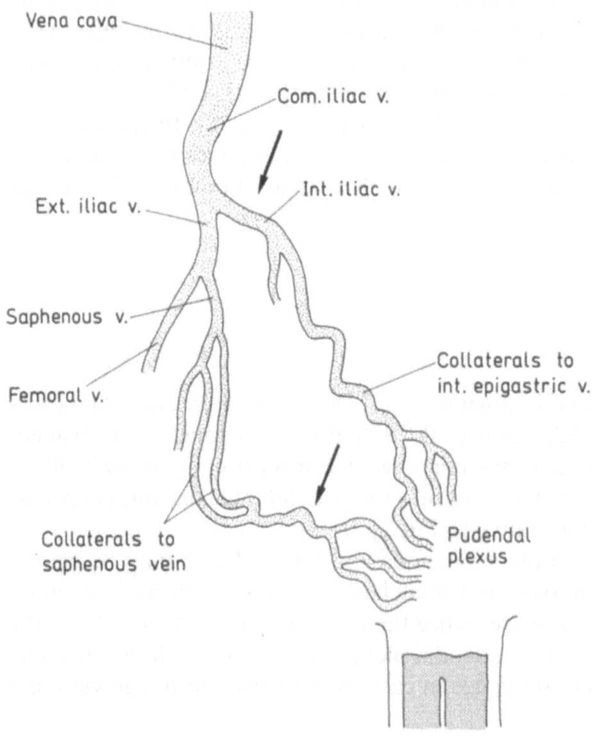

Fig. 2. Venous collaterals for drainage of the corpora cavernosa. *Arrows* indicate location of vein ligations

We made a suprapubic Pfannenstiel incision, split the rectus muscle longitudinally, and exposed the iliac vessels retroperitoneally. The internal iliac vein was dissected at its origin from the common iliac vein and ligated there on both sides. The maintenance flow for an artificial erection was recorded after iliac vein ligation and compared with the preoperative maintenance index.

Results

During the last 3 years, we performed ligation of both internal iliac veins in 52 patients following an exact diagnosis of increased venous drainage (Wagenknecht 1988). The average age of these 52 men was 58 years (range 33–72). In 32 of these men, this procedure was combined with ligation of collaterals to the saphenous and femoral veins from an incision at the penile base. There was a marked improvement of erectile capacity in 36 men (70%). Vein ligation alone was sufficient for an improvement in 26 of them (50%), with an average follow-up of 8 months. In six patients, nitroglycerin spray was additionally used locally on the glans penis in order to improve erectile quality. In four patients with negative papaverine tests preoperatively, iliac vein ligation permitted strong erections after 25 mg papaverine injected intracavernously. In three of these patients, satisfactory erections have occurred lately in between papaverine injections.

Discussion

Internal iliac vein ligation was unsuccessful in 16 of 52 patients (30%). In 10 of these 16 patients, diabetes mellitus was the probable additional cause of neuroarterial lesions. In all patients, the nitroglycerin test showed a one- to sixfold improvement of the inflow through the dorsal and deep penile artery in comparison to preoperative values. This is probably linked to the venous pooling effect of nitroglycerin (Wagenknecht 1988). If there is increased venous drainage, nitroglycerin should only be tried after vein ligation. In 23 of the 52 patients, the preoperative papaverine test was negative or only resulted in weak penile tumescence; postoperatively, the test was positive with two exceptions. In these two patients, an additional cavernous leak was probable (glans appearance time was 38 and 40 s respectively, with an intracavernous flow of 100 ml/min). In cases of increased venous drainage, papaverine/phentolamine therapy should only be used *after* internal iliac vein ligation. The long-term results will show whether this ligation procedure is of value in the treatment of increased venous drainage.

The combination of venous collaterals and cavernous leaks into the glans/corpus spongiosum should be treated by prostheses. We also consider most diabetics who suffer from neurovascular impotence to be candidates for penile prostheses (Wagenknecht et al. 1981). For combined arteriovenous insufficiency, arterialization of the penis with saphenous vein grafts and additional vein ligation was performed in four patients. In this situation, the internal iliac veins should be ligated first. Thereafter, the flow rate necessary to maintain an artificial erection should be determined, and the length (and hence the caliber!) of the saphenous vein graft used for penile arterialization should be adjusted accordingly.

References

Buvat J, Lemaire A, Buvat-Herbaut M, Dehaene JL, Marcolin G (1986) Erectile impotence with venous incompetence: extensive study of 64 cases. Proceedings of the 2nd World Meeting on Impotence, Prague, 1986, University Press, Prague

Duncan JA (1895) Old age – a myth. Toledo Med Surg Rep 8:163

Lewis RW, Puyau FA, Bell DP (1986) Another surgical approach for vasculogenic impotence. J Urol 136:1210

Lue FF, Zeineh SL, Schmidt RA, Tanago EA (1983) Physiology of penile erection. World J Urol 1:194

Lydston GF (1908) The surgical treatment of impotency. Amer J Clin Med 15:1571

Porst H, Ahlen J (1986) Flowmetrical and cavernosometrical studies in potent and impotent men – report on 140 cases. Proceedings of the 2nd World Meeting on Impotence, Prague, 1986

Richard DJ (1982) Anatomy, physiology and neurophysiology of male sexual function. In: Bennet AH (ed) Management of male impotence. Williams and Wilkins, Baltimore

Stief CG (1986) Suggestion for classification of venous leakage. Proceedings of the 2nd World Meeting on Impotence, Prague, 1986

Tudoriu T (1986) The importance of the sclerosis of the corpora cavernosa. Proceedings of the 2nd World Meeting of Impotence, Prague, 1986

Virag R (1985) Human penile erection. J Urol 133:191

Wagenknecht LV (1988) Impotenz: Pathophysiologie – Diagnostik – Therapie. Diesbach, Berlin

Wagenknecht LV, Shukfeh F (1986) Value of infusion-cavernosography for diagnosis of erectile lesions. Proceedings of the 2nd World Meeting of Impotence, Prague, 1986

Wagenknecht LV, Furlow WL, Auvert J (1981) Genitourinary reconstruction with prostheses. Thieme-Stratton, New York

Wagner G (1984) Vascular mechanisms involved in human erection. Int Angiol 3:221

Wespes E, Schulman CC (1985) Venous leakage: surgical treatment of a curable cause of impotence. J Urol 133:796

Wooten JS (1902) Ligation of the dorsal vein of the penis as a cure for atonic impotence. Texas Med J 18:325

Subject Index

W. Eicher, Mannheim;
G. Kockott; H.-J. Vogt,
Munich (Eds.)

Sexology

1988. 72 figures. 133 tables. Approx. 350 pages. Soft cover. ISBN 3-540-19400-2

Sexology as a discipline has had to fight for full-fledged recognition in the scientific community. Yet special knowledge of normal and disturbed sexual behavior is expected of medical professionals, psychologists and educators alike.

Based on the papers given at the 8th World Congress for Sexology in 1987, this volume gives an up-to-date discussion of the most interesting and controversial topics, such as AIDS, in the field. Contributions have been grouped under the main headings: Family Planning, Sterility and Sexuality, Erectile Dysfunction, Sexuality in the Elderly and in Marriage, Transsexualism, Sexual Therapy, and Sexuality and Illness and include items of historical interest as well as trans-cultural comparisons.

Springer-Verlag
Berlin Heidelberg New York
London Paris Tokyo Hong Kong

B. Runnebaum, T. Rabe, L. Kiesel, Heidelberg (Eds.)

Female Contraception

Update and Trends

1988. 83 figures. 90 tables. Approx. 350 pages. Soft cover. ISBN 3-540-19396-0

Contraceptives have always provided ground for controversy. This book describes and discusses latest findings concerning the advantages as well as hazard and risk factors of contraception.

The clinical impact of oral contraceptives on metabolism is particularly highlighted. In addition, behavioural methods, intrauterine devices, implants and modern approaches in animal and clinical research in the field of immunization against pregnancy are considered.

Last, but not least, the book summarizes the complex ethical, religious and political aspects of family planning and contraception.

Springer-Verlag
Berlin Heidelberg New York
London Paris Tokyo Hong Kong

Springer

MIX
Papier aus verantwortungsvollen Quellen
Paper from responsible sources
FSC® C105338

If you have any concerns about our products,
you can contact us on
ProductSafety@springernature.com

In case Publisher is established outside the EU,
the EU authorized representative is:
Springer Nature Customer Service Center GmbH
Europaplatz 3, 69115 Heidelberg, Germany

Printed by Libri Plureos GmbH
in Hamburg, Germany